Copyright © Aiden Blake 2023

All rights reserved.

No part of this book may be reproduced in any form or by any electronic or mechanical means, including information storage and retrieval systems, without written permission from the author, except for the use of brief quotations in a book review.

DISCLAIMER AND LEGAL NOTICE

The information provided in this book is intended for informational purposes only. It is not to be used as a substitute for professional advice or treatment. The author and publisher disclaim any liability arising directly or indirectly from the use of this book.

While every effort has been made to ensure the accuracy of the content, the author and publisher make no guarantees or warranties, express or implied, about the completeness, accuracy, or reliability of the information contained herein.

You should consult with a professional where appropriate. The author and publisher shall not be liable for any loss of profit or any other damages, including but not limited to special, incidental, consequential, or other damages.

CONTENTS

Introduction   vii

1. AWAKENING YOUR GUT-BRAIN AXIS   1
   The Science of Gut-Brain Communication: Understanding the signals   3
   Mood and Food: How your diet affects your emotions   5
   Mindful Practices: Techniques to synchronize your gut and brain for optimal health   7

2. CULTIVATING YOUR INNER GARDEN   21
   Planting the Seeds: Choosing the right foods for a flourishing microbiome   22
   Weeding Out Harmful Habits: Identifying and eliminating gut health disruptors   29
   Nourishing Your Microbiome: Lifestyle choices that promote microbial diversity   40

3. THE ENZYMATIC EDGE   52
   The Role of Enzymes in Digestion: How enzymes work to break down food   58
   Identifying Enzyme Insufficiency: Symptoms and solutions   60
   Enhancing Your Enzymatic Activity: Foods and habits that boost your enzyme power   63

4. FORTIFYING YOUR IMMUNE FORTRESS   67
   The Immune System's Command Center: The gut's role in immunity   68
   Allies in Immunity: Probiotics and their contribution to your defense system   74
   Lifestyle Immune Boosters: Daily practices to strengthen your immune response   78

5. PURIFYING YOUR GUT — 84
The Detoxification Pathways in Your Gut: How your body naturally detoxifies — 85
Supporting Your Body's Cleansing Efforts: Foods and habits that aid detox — 91
Signs of a Clogged Gut: How to tell if your detox pathways need support — 93

6. MOVEMENT FOR MOMENTUM — 100
Physical Activity and Your Digestive System: The connection between exercise and gut function — 101
Types of Movement for Optimal Gut Health: Tailoring your exercise routine — 109
Building a Sustainable Movement Habit: Strategies for long-term success — 121

7. SOOTHING THE EMOTIONAL GUT — 123
Understanding the Impact of Stress and Emotions: The science of emotional digestion — 124
Tactics for Emotional Regulation: Methods to manage stress and its digestive repercussions — 128
The Art of Mindful Eating: How to enhance digestion through mindfulness — 133

8. RESTORATIVE REST FOR DIGESTIVE HEALTH — 144
The Sleep-Digestion Connection: Exploring the impact of sleep on the gut — 145
Sleep Hygiene for Gut Harmony: Best practices for restful sleep — 156
Addressing Sleep Disorders: Approaches to managing sleep issues for digestive benefits — 159

9. BALANCING THE MICROBIOME — 164
Microbiome Analysis: Understanding the state of your gut flora — 165
Dietary Interventions: Adjusting your diet to rebalance the microbiome — 175

10. **INTEGRATING HOLISTIC PRACTICES** 182
   Beyond Diet and Exercise: Exploring additional
   practices 183
   The Supplement Strategy: How to effectively
   incorporate supplements 192
   The Power of Routine: Establishing a holistic
   routine for lifelong gut health 203

   Epilogue 210

   Review Request 213
   Bibliography 217
   About the Author 225

INTRODUCTION

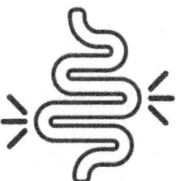

Life, as we know it, can take unexpected turns. Struggles with weight gain, low energy, and emotional turmoil have become a constant in my life. The solution, it turned out, wasn't in the latest fad diet or the most rigorous workout regime, but in my gut. My journey towards gut health not only revolutionized my physical being but also brought about an emotional metamorphosis.

Our bodies are an intricate network of systems working in harmony, with one unlikely hero at the center - our gut. This

INTRODUCTION

isn't just a personal revelation, but a scientifically-backed truth that has come to light in recent years. As someone who has experienced the transformative power of optimal gut health firsthand, I am here to share my story and guide you on a journey towards digestive harmony.

THE GUT AS THE CORNERSTONE OF HEALTH

Our gut is not just an organ of digestion, it's the command center of our overall well-being. This guide adopts a holistic approach that views the gut as the cornerstone of health, affecting everything from our weight to our emotional state. Understanding the gut's intricate workings and its symbiotic relationship with the rest of our body can unlock the secret to lasting health and vitality. I aim to guide you on that enlightening journey.

When we talk about gut health, we're not just talking about avoiding stomach aches. We're talking about the pivotal role it plays in our overall health.

A study published in the Journal of Translational Medicine shows a strong link between gut health and various body systems, including the immune and nervous systems. This guide takes a holistic approach to health, with the gut at its core, affecting everything from your energy levels to your weight and emotional well-being.

Some key aspects we'll delve into include:

- The gut-brain axis and its role in mental health
- How gut health influences metabolism and weight management

- The gut's role in maintaining a strong immune system

DECODING THE GUT-HEALTH MYTHOLOGY

The realm of gut health is fraught with myths and misinformation that can lead one astray. Along our journey together, we will debunk these myths, providing scientific and evidence-based insights into gut health. It's time to separate fact from fiction and gain a clear, lucid understanding of your body's most influential organ.

The world of gut health is riddled with myths and misunderstandings. From oversimplified diet recommendations to complex scientific terms taken out of context, these myths can be misleading and potentially harmful.

We'll debunk common misconceptions such as:

- The idea that all bacteria in your gut are harmful
- The notion that a single diet plan can suit everyone's gut health needs
- The myth that gut health only affects digestion

NAVIGATING THE 10 STEPS

This book serves as a roadmap, guiding you through a 10-step process to achieve digestive harmony and reap benefits for your body and mind. Each step is meticulously detailed, with actionable advice, practical exercises, and essential knowledge about your gut.

Whether you're looking to boost your energy levels, manage

INTRODUCTION

your weight, or enhance your emotional well-being, these steps will lead you toward your objective, one digestible bite at a time. Prepare to embark on this transformative journey towards optimal gut health and overall wellness.

Through the ten steps, you'll:

- Learn to identify signs of poor gut health
- Understand the role of gut-friendly foods and how to incorporate them into your diet
- Discover the link between stress management and gut health
- Gain tools to maintain gut health for long-term benefits

1
AWAKENING YOUR GUT-BRAIN AXIS

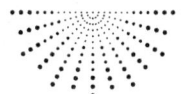

The human gut, often referred to as the 'second brain' due to its intricate connection with our central nervous system, is not just a simple digestive tract. It's a bustling metropolis of trillions of microorganisms, including bacteria, viruses, fungi, and other microbes. This microbiome, as it's called, aids in the digestion of food, the production of vitamins and plays a vital role in our immune system.

Interestingly, the gut houses about 70% of our immune cells, making it a frontline defense against many diseases. It also produces around 90% of the body's serotonin, a neurotransmitter that affects mood, sleep, appetite, and digestion. With this in mind, it's easy to see how you can swiftly and negatively agitate your sleeping patterns, desire to eat and digest in comfort when you treat your gut poorly, effecting the production of Serotonin.

The gut-brain connection, or the gut-brain axis as it's often referred to, is a bidirectional communication system that links the emotional and cognitive centers of the brain with peripheral intestinal functions. This connection suggests that the state of our gut can influence our mental health.

Scientific research has uncovered fascinating facts supporting this connection. For example, a study published in the Journal of Psychiatric Research in 2020 found a significant correlation between gut microbiota composition and depression. Another study from the American Gastroenterological Association found that people with irritable bowel syndrome (IBS) show abnormalities in the gut-brain interaction, leading to the disorder's physical and mental symptoms.

Furthermore, the gut can affect our energy levels and weight management. Gut microbes help break down complex carbohydrates, producing short-chain fatty acids, which are a significant energy source for the body. They also influence how we store fat, how we balance glucose levels, and how we respond to hormones that make us feel hungry or full.

The good news is that we can improve our gut health through diet and lifestyle. Consuming a diet rich in fiber, fruits, vegetables, lean proteins, and healthy fats can foster a healthy gut microbiome. Regular exercise, adequate sleep, and stress management techniques such as meditation also contribute positively to gut health.

Understanding the gut's complexity and its influence on our overall health is not only a fascinating scientific journey but also a practical guide to healthier living. By nurturing our 'second brain,' we can potentially improve our physical health, mental well-being, and overall quality of life.

THE SCIENCE OF GUT-BRAIN COMMUNICATION: UNDERSTANDING THE SIGNALS

The gut-brain axis, a term coined to describe the two-way communication between our digestive system and the brain, is a crucial component of our body's overall function. This axis isn't just a metaphorical highway for messages to travel from our gut to our brain, but a physical and biochemical network involving our nervous system, hormones, and immune system.

At the heart of this communication are neurotransmitters, biochemical messengers that play key roles in our body's physiological responses, including mood, appetite, and digestion. A prime example is serotonin, often called the 'happy chemical,' due to its significant role in mood regulation. As previously mentioned, up to 90% of serotonin is produced in the gut, highlighting the profound impact of gut health on our emotional state.

Another key player in this communication is the vagus nerve, the longest cranial nerve that acts as a two-way information superhighway between the brain and the gut. The vagus nerve transmits signals about the state of the gut's microbiome to the brain, and vice versa, allowing for a constant exchange of information.

Hormones, too, are essential in this dialogue. Ghrelin, often referred to as the 'hunger hormone,' is produced in the stomach and signals the brain when it's time to eat. Meanwhile, leptin, produced by fat cells, tells the brain when we're full.

In addition, cytokines, a type of protein involved in cell signaling, play a crucial role in gut-brain communication. They can affect brain function, influencing feelings of fatigue and depression. Interestingly, certain types of gut bacteria can influence cytokine levels, reinforcing the importance of a healthy gut microbiome.

Understanding these complex interactions between the gut and the brain can provide significant insights into our health and well-being. For instance, imbalances in the gut microbiome, termed dysbiosis, have been linked to a variety of conditions, including obesity, anxiety, depression, and even neurodegenerative diseases like Parkinson's.

By nurturing our gut health through balanced nutrition, regular exercise, adequate sleep, and stress management, we can potentially optimize this communication, supporting not only our digestive health but also our mental well-being and overall health. The science of gut-brain communication is a burgeoning field, and its future findings promise to provide even more profound insights into human health.

here is a list of key signals involved in the gut-brain communication:

- **Neurotransmitters**: These biochemical messengers play a critical role in our body's physiological responses. A prime example is serotonin, often called the 'happy chemical,' due to its significant role in mood regulation. Most of our body's serotonin is produced in the gut.
- **Vagus Nerve**: This is the longest cranial nerve in our body, acting as a two-way information superhighway between the brain and the gut. It transmits signals about the state of the gut's microbiome to the brain, and vice versa.

- **Hormones**: Hormones also play a crucial role in this communication. Ghrelin, the 'hunger hormone,' is produced in the stomach and signals the brain when it's time to eat. Leptin, on the other hand, is produced by fat cells and tells the brain when we're full.
- **Cytokines**: These are a type of protein involved in cell signaling. They can affect brain function, influencing feelings of fatigue and depression. Certain types of gut bacteria can influence cytokine levels, further emphasizing the importance of a healthy gut microbiome.

By understanding these signals and how they interact, we can gain significant insights into our health and well-being. Nurturing our gut health can potentially optimize this communication, supporting not only our digestive health but also our mental well-being and overall health.

MOOD AND FOOD: HOW YOUR DIET AFFECTS YOUR EMOTIONS

Often, we think of food merely as fuel for our bodies, providing the energy we need to power through the day but did you know that what we eat can also significantly impact our emotions and mental health? That's right, our dietary choices can affect our mood, stress levels, and even our cognitive function.

This connection comes down to the gut-brain axis because of the vital role it plays in producing neurotransmitters, chemicals that help regulate our mood.

One of the key players in this process is our gut microbiome, an ecosystem of trillions of bacteria, viruses, and fungi that live in our digestive tract. Our diet shapes this microbiome, and in turn, these microbes impact our emotions.

For instance, fermented foods and those rich in probiotics—like yogurt, kimchi, and kefir—can positively influence our mood. These foods boost beneficial gut bacteria that can produce neurotransmitters like serotonin, gamma-aminobutyric acid (GABA), and dopamine, known to enhance our mood and cognitive function. Moreover, they can decrease inflammation, a factor linked to many mood disorders.

On the other hand, A diet predominantly consisting of processed foods, saturated fats, and sugars can significantly alter the composition and function of the gut microbiota, leading to a condition referred to as dysbiosis. Dysbiosis is characterized by an imbalance in the microbial community in the gut, where beneficial bacteria are diminished, and potentially harmful bacteria become more prevalent. This shift can impair the gut barrier function, leading to an increased permeability, often referred to as "leaky gut," and result in systemic inflammation.

So, how can we use this knowledge to nourish our bodies and minds? Firstly, by incorporating a variety of nutrient-rich foods into our diet—plenty of fruits, vegetables, whole grains, lean proteins, and healthy fats. Secondly, reducing the intake of processed foods, which can negatively impact our gut health and, consequently, our mood.

Remember our diet doesn't just feed our bodies, it also feeds our emotions. So next time you're planning your meals, consider not just what your body needs, but also what your mind might benefit from. This understanding of the food-mood connection offers a powerful tool for enhancing our emotional well-being and overall health.

Here's a simplified chart illustrating how certain foods are linked to our moods.

Foods	Linked Mood
Fermented Foods (yogurt, kefir, kimchi, sauerkraut, tempeh)	Beneficial for mood and cognitive function. These foods boost 'good' gut bacteria, which produce mood-enhancing neurotransmitters.
Omega-3 Fatty Acids (salmon, mackerel, chia seeds, flaxseeds, walnuts)	Helpful for brain health and mood regulation. Omega-3 fatty acids can reduce inflammation and help produce neurotransmitters.
Whole Grains (brown rice, oatmeal, quinoa)	Good for steady energy and mood. Whole grains have a low glycemic index, preventing blood sugar spikes and crashes that can affect mood.
Leafy Greens (spinach, kale, swiss chard)	Rich in folate and other B vitamins, which are linked to the production of serotonin, a mood-enhancing neurotransmitter.
Berries (blueberries, strawberries, raspberries)	High in antioxidants, which can reduce inflammation and boost mood.
Dark Chocolate	Can boost mood and reduce stress. It contains phenylethylamine, which encourages your brain to release feel-good endorphins.
Processed Foods (fast food, sugary drinks, snacks)	Can disrupt gut health and lead to mood swings, anxiety, and depression.
Alcohol	Can disrupt sleep patterns, lead to mood swings, and exacerbate symptoms of anxiety and depression.

MINDFUL PRACTICES: TECHNIQUES TO SYNCHRONIZE YOUR GUT AND BRAIN FOR OPTIMAL HEALTH

Mindfulness practices such as meditation and yoga are not just beneficial for the mind, but also for the body – specifically, the gut. The intricate connection between the gut and the brain is significantly influenced by these practices.

Consider this: a study published in the "Journal of Clinical Psychology" revealed that an 8-week mindfulness-based stress reduction (MBSR) program led to significant reductions in inflammatory markers. This is crucial as inflammation often signals a distressed gut. By mitigating inflammation, mindfulness practices can contribute to better gut health, and by extension, overall wellbeing.

Similarly, yoga, too, has been found to contribute to improved gut health. Research published in the "International Journal of Yoga" highlighted that regular yoga practice can help maintain a healthy gut microbiota composition. A balanced gut microbiota is critically important for our overall health, helping with digestion, the production of essential vitamins, and even the regulation of our immune system.

The influence of mindfulness extends beyond gut health to our eating habits. The practice of mindful eating, which involves being fully present and aware during eating, has been associated with healthier eating habits and improved digestive health.

In a study published in "Eating Behaviors", individuals who engage in mindful eating were found to be less likely to binge eat, have healthier body weight, and experience fewer depressive symptoms. By being fully present in the moment, individuals can better recognize their body's hunger and fullness cues, make healthier food choices, and find greater enjoyment in eating.

Mindful Meditation

Mindful meditation is a practice that involves focusing your mind on the present moment, and accepting it without judgment. This practice is known to reduce stress and anxiety, which can have a direct impact on your gut health. Chronic stress can disrupt the balance of your gut microbiota, leading to digestive issues. By reducing stress, mindful meditation can help restore this balance, improving overall gut health.

A simple mindful meditation practice could be setting aside 10-15 minutes each day in a quiet space. During this time, focus on your breath going in and out.

Yoga

Yoga is a physical, mental, and spiritual practice that combines breath control, meditation, and movement. Specific yoga poses can help stimulate digestion by increasing blood flow to the digestive tract, stimulating the intestines, and helping food move through the system. This is quite similar to how the Japanese and other Asian cultures position themselves when using squat toilets, which are designed to allow natural posture for the human body during defecation but we won't delve into detail on this one right now.

Poses such as the Seated Forward Bend (Paschimottanasana), the Supine Spinal Twist (Supta Matsyendrasana), and the Knees-to-Chest pose (Apanasana) are particularly beneficial for digestive health. It's important to remember, though, that yoga should be practiced under the guidance of a certified instructor to ensure the poses are done correctly and safely.

- **Aids Digestion:** Certain yoga poses, such as the Pavanamuktasana (Wind Relieving Pose), Apanasana (Knees-to-Chest Pose), and Malasana (Garland Pose or Squat), mimic the natural squatting position, promoting the expulsion of gas and facilitating bowel movements.

- **Stimulates Organs:** Many yoga poses involve twisting the torso, which massages abdominal organs, stimulating digestion and helping to detoxify the body. Poses like Ardha Matsyendrasana (Half Lord of the Fishes Pose) and Marichyasana (Marichi's Pose) are examples of such twists.
- •**Reduces Stress:** Yoga practices are known to reduce stress and anxiety through mindful breathing and relaxation techniques. Since stress can negatively impact gut health, leading to issues like irritable bowel syndrome (IBS), the calming effect of yoga on the nervous system can indirectly benefit gut health.

Mindful Eating

Mindful eating as briefly discussed is the practice of paying attention to your food and your body's response to it. It involves eating slowly, without distraction, savoring every bite, and listening to your body's cues for hunger and fullness.

When you eat mindfully, you are more likely to consume the right amount of food, not overeating, which can stress the digestive system. You become more aware of the foods that nourish you and those that don't, leading to better food choices.

The practice of mindful eating can start with small steps such as removing distractions during meal times, taking smaller bites, chewing thoroughly, and taking time to appreciate the colors, smells, and textures of your food. Chewing is the first step in the digestive process, and it has several important functions that facilitate digestion and absorption of nutrients in the gut. Here's why mindful eating and thorough chewing are important:

- **Saliva Production and Enzymatic Breakdown:** Chewing stimulates the production of saliva, which contains enzymes such as amylase and lipase that begin the chemical breakdown of food. Amylase starts the digestion of carbohydrates by breaking down starch into simpler sugars, while lipase initiates the digestion of fats. Mindful eating encourages slower, more thorough chewing, which allows these enzymes more time to act on the food, leading to better digestion.
- **Physical Breakdown of Food:** Chewing breaks the food into smaller particles, increasing the surface area available for digestive enzymes to work. This physical breakdown is crucial for the efficient extraction of nutrients as the food passes through the digestive tract. By practicing mindful eating and focusing on chewing, you ensure that food is adequately broken down before it reaches the stomach and intestines, easing the work required from the rest of the digestive system.
- **Enhances Absorption:** The more thoroughly the food is chewed, the easier it becomes for the body to absorb nutrients. Large, poorly chewed food particles are harder for the body to break down and can pass through the gut without fully releasing their nutrients. Mindful eating helps prevent this by

ensuring food is well-chewed and ready for optimal nutrient extraction.

Deep Breathing Exercises

Deep breathing exercises, sometimes known as diaphragmatic breathing, involve inhaling deeply into the diaphragm rather than shallow breathing into the chest. This kind of breathing activates the body's relaxation response, leading to a state of calmness.

The relaxation response can aid in digestion as stress and anxiety have been linked to disruption in the gut microbiota. By reducing stress through deep breathing, we can promote better gut health.

You can make use of proven breathing techniques such as the box breathing technique, also known as square breathing or four-square breathing, which is a simple yet powerful relaxation method that can help manage stress, improve concentration, and enhance overall well-being. This technique involves four main steps, each lasting for an equal duration, traditionally four seconds. The process is visualized as the four sides of a box, hence the name. Here's how to do it:

- **Inhale:** Begin by slowly exhaling to empty your lungs. Then, gently inhale through your nose to a slow count of four, filling your lungs with air. Visualize drawing a line up one side of a square as you count.
- **Hold:** Hold your breath for another count of four. Imagine drawing a line across the top of the square.

This pause allows oxygen to fully saturate your bloodstream.
- **Exhale:** Slowly exhale through your mouth for a count of four, emptying the lungs. As you exhale, visualize drawing a line down the other side of the square. This helps to remove carbon dioxide and other waste gases from your body.
- **Hold Again:** Hold your breath for a final count of four, completing the square by drawing the bottom line. This pause eliminates residual air from the lungs and prepares you for the next breath.

Repeat this cycle for several minutes, or as long as needed to feel its calming effects. Box breathing is beneficial for calming the mind, reducing stress, and improving focus and concentration. It can be practiced anywhere and anytime you need to find calm or prepare for a stressful situation. The simplicity of box breathing makes it accessible to anyone, including those new to breathwork or meditation practices.

When your mind wanders, as it naturally will, gently bring your focus back to your breath without judgment, and over time it will become second nature.

Regular Physical Exercise

Regular physical exercise is crucial for maintaining a healthy gut. Exercise increases the efficiency of the digestive system, helping to speed up the movement of food through it, which can be beneficial for those suffering from constipation or bloating.

Furthermore, physical activity has been shown to increase the diversity of gut bacteria which is linked to better overall health. Exercise can be as simple as a daily walk, or more strenuous activities like running, swimming, or weightlifting, depending on your fitness level and preference. here are suggestions for different forms of exercise that you can utilize with ease:

- **Daily Walking:** A simple yet effective form of exercise, walking for at least 30 minutes a day can stimulate digestion and support gut health. It's accessible, requires no equipment, and can be easily integrated into your daily routine.
- **Pilates:** These forms of exercise are particularly beneficial for the digestive system, as many poses and movements specifically target the abdominal area, encouraging movement through the digestive tract and helping to relieve gas and bloating.
- **Aerobic Exercises:** Activities such as running, cycling, and swimming increase heart rate and blood flow, which in turn can enhance gut motility and promote the growth of beneficial gut bacteria. These can be adapted to fit your fitness level and preferences.
- **Strength Training:** Engaging in resistance or weightlifting exercises a few times a week can improve overall body composition, which indirectly supports gut health by reducing fat mass and inflammation.

- **Outdoor Activities:** Activities like hiking, kayaking, or team sports not only provide physical exercise but also exposure to diverse environments, which may contribute to a more varied gut microbiota.

Probiotic and Prebiotic Foods

Probiotics are beneficial bacteria that can help maintain a healthy balance in your gut microbiota, while prebiotics are types of dietary fiber that feed these good bacteria.

Probiotic-rich foods include yogurt, sauerkraut, kimchi, and other fermented foods. These foods can help replenish beneficial bacteria in your gut, aiding in digestion and overall gut health.

Prebiotic foods, on the other hand, include bananas, oats, apples, and other high-fiber foods. These foods provide nourishment for the beneficial bacteria, allowing them to thrive and maintain a healthy balance.

Consuming a mix of both probiotic and prebiotic foods can help ensure your gut microbiota remains balanced, leading to better digestion and overall health.

Adequate Sleep

Adequate sleep is a cornerstone for overall health, including that of your gut. There's a bidirectional relationship between sleep and your gut. While poor gut health can lead to sleep disturbances, lack of good quality sleep can also disturb the gut-brain axis, leading to an imbalance in the gut bacteria.

It's generally recommended to aim for 7-9 hours of sleep

per night. Establishing a regular sleep schedule, creating a comfortable sleep environment, and avoiding screens before bed can all contribute to better sleep quality.

As a parent, it is essential to acknowledge that achieving uninterrupted periods of rest or personal time can be challenging and often unrealistic, particularly depending on the age and needs of your child. In many cases, the most feasible approach to rest is to capitalize on the opportunities provided by your child's nap times.

Reducing Intake of Processed Foods

Processed foods often contain additives and preservatives that can negatively impact the balance of your gut bacteria. They're also often high in unhealthy fats and sugars, and low in fiber, which is important for gut health.

By reducing the intake of processed foods and incorporating more whole, unprocessed foods into your diet such as fruits, vegetables, lean proteins, and whole grains, you can help maintain a healthy gut. These foods are not only higher in fiber but also contain a variety of nutrients that support gut health.

Hydration

Staying properly hydrated is fundamental for overall health, playing a pivotal role in various bodily functions, including the maintenance of gut health. Water facilitates the digestion of food and the absorption of nutrients by dissolving fats and soluble fiber, allowing these substances to pass more easily through the intestines. Moreover, adequate hydration is essential for the mucosal lining of the intestines, which acts as a barrier against harmful substances and bacteria, thereby maintaining intestinal integrity.

Water also helps in the proliferation of beneficial gut bacteria, contributing to a balanced microbiome, which is crucial for digestion, the synthesis of certain vitamins, and the immune system.

While the "8 glasses of water a day" rule is a commonly cited guideline, the actual amount of water needed can vary significantly among individuals. Factors influencing hydration needs include age, sex, weight, physical activity level, and environmental conditions.

The Institute of Medicine suggests a daily intake of about 3.7 liters (about 125 ounces) for men and 2.7 liters (about 91 ounces) for women from all beverages and foods. Given that about 20% of our fluid intake typically comes from food, this translates to an approximate goal of 9 cups of fluids a day for women and 13 cups for men.

Remember that the quality of the water you use to hydrate is just as important and can be a big difference. For example, tap water can vary depending on the source and the treatment processes it undergoes but contaminants such as heavy metals, chlorine, pesticides, and microorganisms can sometimes be found in tap water, posing health risks. Chronic exposure to certain contaminants can lead to gastrointestinal and other health issues so it would be beneficial to your gut to consider the following options.

- **Filters:** Look for filters that can remove specific contaminants present in your local water supply.

Activated carbon filters, reverse osmosis, and ion exchange filters are popular options.
- **Distillation:** A process that involves boiling water and then condensing the steam back into water. This method removes minerals and impurities but also demineralizes the water, which may necessitate adding minerals back for taste and health benefits.

Stress Management

Stress management is a crucial element for optimal gut health. Chronic stress doesn't just affect your mental state, it can also lead to physical changes in the body, including the gut. Prolonged stress can disrupt the balance of bacteria in your gut, impair the immune response, and lead to inflammation, all of which can contribute to various gut problems such as irritable bowel syndrome (IBS), stomach ulcers, and more.

While deep breathing, yoga, and meditation are excellent techniques for managing stress, there are other approaches you can consider:

- **Progressive Muscle Relaxation (PMR):** This technique involves tensing and then releasing different muscle groups in the body. It's a way to physically relax your body, which can, in turn, improve mental relaxation as well.

- **Mindfulness:** This practice involves focusing your attention on the present moment, and accepting it without judgment. Mindfulness can be practiced

through simple acts like mindful eating, where you pay attention to each bite, savor it, and observe your reactions to the food without judgment. This can help reduce stress and also improve your relationship with food.
- **Therapy and Counseling**: If stress is consistently high, speaking with a mental health professional can be beneficial. Therapies like cognitive-behavioral therapy (CBT) can provide you with effective strategies to manage and reduce stress.
- **Leisure Activities**: Engaging in activities you enjoy can help reduce stress. This could be anything from reading a book, painting, gardening, or going for a walk in nature. These activities can divert your mind from stressors and provide a sense of relaxation and happiness.

Remember, everyone's experience with stress is different, and so the most effective stress management techniques can vary. It's about finding what works best for you and integrating it into your lifestyle to promote both mental and gut health.

Each of these practices individually contributes to a healthier gut-brain connection, and when combined, they can significantly contribute to overall health and well-being.

As we transition now to our next chapter, it is important to consider these practices as essential tools for nurturing our inner garden. This metaphorical garden represents our gut health, a delicate ecosystem that requires regular care and attention.

In the next chapter, we will delve deeper into how mindfulness practices and mindful eating can help us cultivate a thriving inner garden. We will explore practical exercises and provide detailed guides on how to incorporate these practices into our daily routines.

From understanding the importance of balanced gut microbiota to learning how to respond mindfully to our body's cues, our goal is to equip you with the knowledge and tools needed to nurture your inner garden, enhancing not just your gut health, but your overall well-being.

2
CULTIVATING YOUR INNER GARDEN

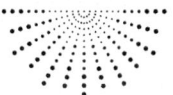

The doctor of the future will give no medication but will interest his patients in the care of the human frame, diet and in the cause and prevention of disease.

— THOMAS EDISON

In our previous discussions, we've unearthed the significance of our gut health and how mindfulness practices can cultivate a flourishing gut ecosystem. Now, picture this - your gut is a vibrant, bustling garden. Each bacterium, a tiny seedling, together creates a thriving ecosystem that is as diverse and rich as the most bountiful of gardens.

Just as a gardener meticulously tends to each plant, making sure it receives just the right amount of sunlight, water, and nutrients, so too must we tend to our gut flora. Neglect could lead to an overgrowth of harmful bacteria, and weeds in our garden, which can upset the balance and compromise our overall well-being.

Imagine the possibilities when your inner garden is well-tended. A robust immune system, a healthy body weight, improved mood, and enhanced cognitive function are just a few of the benefits that come with a flourishing gut flora ecosystem. However, nurturing this garden is not a one-time event, it's an ongoing commitment, much like the gardener's task.

As we delve into the next chapter, we will explore in detail the ways to tend to this inner garden. We will unravel the science behind gut health, understand the role of diet and lifestyle in shaping our gut flora, and provide practical tips on maintaining a healthy gut microbiota.

We will guide you on this fascinating journey, equip you with the needed knowledge and tools to nurture your inner garden and help you comprehend how to tune into your body's needs.

So, are you ready to roll up your sleeves and start cultivating? The path to a healthier, happier you must begin in your gut, and it's time we started tending to it. Let's get into it then.

PLANTING THE SEEDS: CHOOSING THE RIGHT FOODS FOR A FLOURISHING MICROBIOME

The gut microbiome, much like a complex, diverse garden, requires careful nurturing and the right 'seeds' or inputs - primarily in the form of food, to thrive. Let's delve deeper into how different foods can shape and enhance our gut flora.

Fiber-Rich Foods

Dietary fiber is a vital component of gut health. It functions as a source of nourishment for beneficial gut bacteria like Bifidobacteria and Lactobacilli. As these bacteria ferment the fiber, they produce short-chain fatty acids, which are key players in maintaining the integrity of the gut barrier, reducing inflammation, and promoting overall gut function. The following foods are excellent sources of fiber:

Whole Grains

Whole grains, such as oats, brown rice, quinoa, and whole-grain bread, are rich in dietary fiber. The fiber in whole grains not only nourishes your gut bacteria but also contributes to a feeling of fullness, potentially aiding in weight management.

Fruits and Vegetables

Leafy greens, apples, bananas, berries, carrots, and bell peppers are all fiber powerhouses. These foods provide a variety of fibers and other nutrients, contributing to a diverse and healthy gut microbiota. Plus, the natural sweetness of fruits and the flavors of vegetables can make them a delightful part of your meals.

Legumes

Lentils, chickpeas, and beans are packed with fiber. These foods are not only excellent for gut health but are also a great source of plant-based protein. Incorporating legumes into your diet can support gut health and provide other health benefits like improved blood sugar control, and lower cholesterol.

Remember, while increasing your fiber intake, it's also important to drink plenty of water. Fiber absorbs water in the digestive tract, which can help prevent constipation but can also lead to blockages if not enough water is consumed. So, as you add more fiber to your diet, be sure to stay well-hydrated. Enjoy these fiber-rich foods as part of a balanced diet to keep your gut happy and healthy.

Fermented Foods

Fermented foods are a fantastic addition to our diet. Think of them as robust, healthy plants you're adding to the garden that is your gut. They're rich in probiotics, which are live bacteria that provide health benefits when consumed. These foods can enhance the gut's microbial diversity, helping to outcompete harmful bacteria and restore balance. Here's a closer look:

Yogurt and Kefir

These fermented dairy products are teeming with probiotics, particularly Lactobacillus and Bifidobacterium species. These live cultures can enhance gut health by improving the balance and diversity of the gut microbiota. They also contribute to better digestion and absorption of nutrients, especially lactose, due to their enzymatic activity. Plus, they are often rich in protein and calcium, contributing to overall health.

Sauerkraut and Kimchi

Both of these are fermented cabbage dishes, rich in both probiotics and fiber. The fermentation process increases the availability and digestibility of nutrients, providing a nutritional boost. The probiotics in sauerkraut and kimchi can improve gut health, while the fiber provides nourishment for your gut bacteria. Additionally, these foods are high in vitamin C and other antioxidants, further contributing to health.

While fermented foods are beneficial, they should be consumed as part of a varied and balanced diet. Also, as they can be high in salt, moderation is key. If you are new to fermented foods, start with small amounts to allow your gut to adjust. Your gut is a complex ecosystem, and nourishing it with a diversity of healthy foods, including fermented ones, will help it thrive.

Polyphenol-Rich Foods

Polyphenols are naturally occurring plant compounds that are packed with antioxidant properties, which can aid in reducing inflammation in the body. These compounds also serve as food for the healthy bacteria in your gut, helping them to flourish and outcompete harmful bacteria. Including polyphenol-rich foods in your diet can therefore contribute to a healthier gut. Here's a closer look at some of these foods:

Green Tea

Green tea is a rich source of a specific type of polyphenol known as catechins. These compounds not only have strong antioxidant and anti-inflammatory effects, but they also have a prebiotic effect, promoting the growth of beneficial gut bacteria. Regularly drinking green tea can thus contribute to maintaining a balanced gut microbiota, alongside offering other health benefits like enhanced brain function and fat loss.

Dark Chocolate

Dark chocolate, especially varieties with high cocoa content, is packed with polyphenols. These compounds are metabolized by gut bacteria into anti-inflammatory compounds. In particular, the polyphenols in dark chocolate have been shown to stimulate the growth of Bifidobacteria and Lactobacilli, two types of beneficial bacteria. However, it's important to consume dark chocolate in moderation due to its high-calorie content.

Olive Oil and Berries

Olive oil, particularly extra virgin olive oil, and berries like blueberries, strawberries, and raspberries are also high in polyphenols. These foods can support gut health by increasing the diversity and population of beneficial bacteria in the gut. Additionally, the healthy fats in olive oil and the fiber in berries can further support gut health.

Variety is key to a healthy diet. Incorporating a diverse range of polyphenol-rich foods can help ensure you're nourishing your gut with a broad spectrum of beneficial compounds. Enjoy these foods as part of a balanced diet, and your gut will thank you.

Lean Protein

Protein is an essential part of our diet, and choosing lean sources can contribute positively to gut health. While studies suggest that excessive intake of red and processed meats can negatively impact gut health, lean proteins can be beneficial. These include:

- Fish: Rich in omega-3 fatty acids, fish can reduce inflammation and support gut health.
- Poultry: Chicken and turkey are lean proteins that can be part of a gut-healthy diet.
- Plant-Based Proteins: Foods like lentils, chickpeas, and tofu are not only good protein sources but also rich in fiber.
- Red meat: is rich in essential nutrients that are crucial for body functions. It is a significant source of high-quality protein, which is vital for muscle maintenance and repair. Additionally, red meat contains important vitamins and minerals, including vitamin B12, zinc, and iron. Vitamin B12, found naturally only in animal products, is essential for the production of red blood cells and the maintenance of the central nervous system. Iron from red meat is in the heme form, which is more easily absorbed by the body than non-heme iron

from plant sources, making it crucial in preventing anemia.

Protein digestion, especially comparing plant-based proteins to animal-based proteins, is intriguing and complex. Our bodies process and utilize proteins from various sources differently, due to the nature of the proteins themselves and the other nutrients that accompany them.

Digestibility and Amino Acid Profiles

One of the main differences between animal and plant proteins lies in their digestibility and amino acid profiles. Animal proteins, such as those from meat, dairy, and eggs, are considered "complete" proteins because they contain all nine essential amino acids in proportions that closely match human needs. These proteins are typically more easily digested and absorbed by the body, which means they're readily available for building and repairing tissues, including muscles.

Plant-based proteins, found in foods like lentils, chickpeas, and tofu, while nutritious and beneficial for health, often have a more complex structure and are sometimes referred to as "incomplete" proteins because they may lack one or more of the essential amino acids in sufficient quantities. This doesn't mean plant-based proteins can't meet nutritional needs, but it does mean that a more varied diet is necessary to ensure all amino acid requirements are met.

In essence, a diverse diet leads to a diverse microbiome, which is a cornerstone of gut health. Incorporate these foods into your diet to plant the seeds for a flourishing gut microbiome.

WEEDING OUT HARMFUL HABITS: IDENTIFYING AND ELIMINATING GUT HEALTH DISRUPTORS

To maintain a healthy garden, you must not only plant seeds but also diligently weed out any harmful elements that disrupt the garden's growth and productivity. Similarly, maintaining a healthy gut demands more than just eating a balanced diet; it requires vigilantly identifying and eliminating harmful habits that can disrupt our gut health. Here, we delve into some common detrimental habits, or 'weeds,' that we must guard against:

Excessive Sugar Intake

Sugar, particularly refined sugar, has a reputation for being a major disruptor of our gut health. Consuming sugar in excess can promote the overgrowth of certain types of bacteria and yeast in our gut, creating an imbalance. This condition, known as dysbiosis, can lead to a host of health issues. Here's a closer look:

The science

Overconsumption of sugar can lead to various health problems, such as bloating and inflammation. It can also make us more susceptible to infections. This is because the overgrowth of certain bacteria and yeast can disrupt the balance of our gut microbiota, a key player in our immune function.

The impact

Refined sugar is the main offender. This is the type of sugar that's commonly added to processed foods and beverages. While it can provide a quick energy boost, it offers no nutritional benefits and can have detrimental effects on gut health when consumed in excess.

The Solution

It's crucial to curb excessive sugar intake. Opting for natural sweeteners like fruits, honey, and stevia can be a healthier choice. Fruits, in particular, not only provide natural sweetness but also contain fiber and other nutrients beneficial for gut health. Honey has antimicrobial properties and stevia is a zero-calorie sweetener that doesn't spike blood sugar levels.

Moderation is key when it comes to sugar. Balancing your consumption of sweet foods with a varied and nutrient-dense diet can help maintain a healthy gut microbiota. It's not about eliminating sugar, but about understanding its impact on our health and making mindful choices. Another option is to swap out sugar for sweeteners but they may do more harm than good.

Several artificial sweeteners are widely used today, including aspartame, sucralose, saccharin, and acesulfame potassium. Each has been approved by regulatory agencies like the FDA after undergoing extensive testing. However, despite this approval, some research and public concern have highlighted potential areas of toxicity and adverse effects associated with their consumption:

- **Aspartame**: Found in products like diet sodas, chewing gum, and low-calorie desserts, aspartame has been scrutinized for potential neurological effects, including headaches, migraines, and mood disorders. Some animal studies have suggested a possible link to an increased risk of certain cancers, though comprehensive reviews by regulatory bodies have not found consistent evidence to support a clear risk to human health at normal consumption levels.
- **Sucralose**: Used in baking and in many "sugar-free" products, sucralose is known for its heat stability. Some research has raised concerns about its impact on gut health, including alterations in the microbiome and potential effects on insulin sensitivity and glucose metabolism. However, these findings are not conclusive, and more research is needed to fully understand its long-term implications.
- **Saccharin**: One of the oldest artificial sweeteners, saccharin, has been controversial due to early animal studies linking it to bladder cancer. These results led to it being briefly banned in the 1970s, although subsequent research showed these effects might not be relevant to humans, leading to the ban being lifted and saccharin being declared safe for consumption by the FDA.

- **Acesulfame Potassium**: Often found in soft drinks and mixed with other sweeteners, acesulfame potassium has been criticized for a lack of long-term safety studies. Some animal studies have suggested a potential risk for cancer, but no conclusive evidence has been found to prove a direct link in humans.

Overuse of Antibiotics

Antibiotics are undeniably a medical marvel, playing a pivotal role in combating bacterial infections. But they come with a caveat - they don't distinguish between harmful and beneficial bacteria. Overuse or misuse of these drugs can lead to a significant disruption in our gut flora. Here's a more in-depth look:

The Science

Overuse or misuse of antibiotics can wipe out our beneficial gut bacteria, along with the harmful ones. This can disrupt our gut flora, leading to a condition known as dysbiosis. This imbalance can have a ripple effect on our health, affecting everything from digestion to immunity. This can potentially cause more harm than the infection you are trying to fight.

The Impact

The loss of beneficial bacteria can lead to a host of health issues like digestive problems, increased susceptibility to infections, and even mental health problems, as there is a growing body of research showing a link between gut health and mental health.

The Solution

It's essential to use antibiotics judiciously and only under the guidance of a healthcare provider. Antibiotics should be used when necessary and it's important to complete the full course of the medication as prescribed. Avoiding unnecessary use of antibiotics can help maintain a healthy balance of gut bacteria.

Remember, antibiotics are a powerful tool in the fight against bacterial infections, but they should be used with respect for their potential impact on our gut health. Always consult with a healthcare provider before starting any antibiotic treatment and never self-medicate. A mindful approach to antibiotic use can go a long way in preserving the beneficial bacteria that contribute to our overall well-being.

High-Stress Levels

Our gut, often referred to as our 'second brain,' is intrinsically linked to our mental well-being, thanks to the intricate network of neurons in our gut, known as the enteric nervous system. This system communicates directly with our brain, suggesting a strong connection between our gut health and mental state. Chronic stress, unfortunately, can upset the balance of our gut ecosystem. Here's a more detailed look:

The Science

The enteric nervous system (ENS) is a complex network of neurons that governs the function of the gastrointestinal (GI) tract. Often dubbed the "second brain," the ENS operates autonomously but also communicates extensively with the central nervous system (CNS), which includes the brain and spinal cord.

This communication network incorporates various components, including the ENS, the CNS, the autonomic nervous system (ANS), the hypothalamic-pituitary-adrenal (HPA) axis, and the microbiota residing in the gut.

- **Neural Communication**: The vagus nerve is a key neural pathway in the gut-brain axis, transmitting signals in both directions. For example, changes in the gut's environment can send signals directly to the brain, affecting feelings of hunger or satiety, mood, and stress levels.
- **Hormonal Communication**: The HPA axis, which regulates stress response in the body, is another crucial component. Stress can trigger the HPA axis to release stress hormones like cortisol, which can affect gut permeability, motility, and secretion, as well as the composition of the gut microbiota.
- **Microbiota-Gut-Brain Axis**: The trillions of microbes residing in the gut, collectively known as the microbiota, also play a significant role in the gut-brain axis. These microbes can produce neurotransmitters and metabolites that can cross the

blood-brain barrier, influencing brain function and behavior. They also interact with the immune system, which has its communication network with the brain.

The Impact

The relationship between stress and gut health is a clear demonstration of the gut-brain axis at work. When an individual experiences stress, the brain's response can lead to a cascade of physiological changes in the gut:

- **Altered Gut Motility**: Stress can speed up or slow down the movement of the gastrointestinal tract, leading to symptoms like diarrhea, constipation, or stomach pain.
- **Increased Gut Permeability**: Also known as "leaky gut," this condition allows bacteria and toxins to pass from the gut into the bloodstream, potentially leading to inflammation and other health issues.
- **Changes in Microbiota**: Stress can alter the composition of the gut microbiota, potentially reducing the abundance of beneficial bacteria and increasing harmful bacteria, which can affect both physical and mental health.
- **Immune System Response**: Stress can also modulate the immune system's activity in the gut, leading to inflammation and altered gut function.

The Solution

Incorporating effective stress management techniques into our daily routine is a key factor in maintaining a healthy gut. Regular exercise, meditation, and adequate sleep can help manage stress levels. Exercise not only helps reduce stress but also promotes a healthy gut by encouraging the growth of beneficial bacteria. Meditation can help calm the mind and reduce stress, while adequate sleep is vital for both mental health and gut health.

Remember, maintaining a healthy gut isn't just about what you eat. It's also about how you manage stress. Chronic stress can have a significant impact on your gut health, but by incorporating stress management techniques into your daily routine, you can help maintain a healthy gut ecosystem. It's all about balance and taking a holistic approach to health.

Maintaining a healthy gut is a constant effort of not just nurturing beneficial habits but also actively weeding out harmful ones. By being vigilant of these common disruptors, we can keep our gut flora blooming, thereby improving our overall health and well-being.

here are some techniques that you can make use of and we will discuss others on chapters to come.

- **Social Support**: Connecting with friends, family, or support groups can provide emotional support and reduce stress. Social interactions can trigger the release of oxytocin, a natural stress reliever.
- **Time Management**: Organizing your schedule, setting priorities, and breaking tasks into smaller

steps can help manage stress by making your to-do list more manageable.
- **Hobbies and Interests**: Engaging in activities you enjoy, such as reading, gardening, painting, or playing music, can be a great way to relax and distract yourself from stress.
- **Limiting Screen Time**: Reducing the amount of time spent on electronic devices, especially before bedtime, can help decrease information overload and improve sleep quality.
- **Nature Exposure**: Spending time in nature, whether it's a walk in the park, hiking in the woods, or simply sitting in a garden, can lower stress levels, improve mood, and enhance overall health.
- **Professional Help**: If stress becomes overwhelming, seeking help from a psychologist or counselor can provide strategies to manage stress more effectively. Cognitive-behavioral therapy (CBT) and other therapeutic techniques can be particularly beneficial.

Environmental toxins

In our modern world, the quest for optimal gut health has become increasingly complex, as we navigate through an environment teeming with potential disruptors. Among these, environmental toxins and chemicals stand out as silent assailants, subtly undermining our health through our most basic needs: the air we breathe, the water we drink, and the food we consume. Recognizing and addressing the impact of these toxins is crucial for anyone looking to protect and enhance their gut health.

The Science

Environmental toxins and chemicals, ranging from pesticides and herbicides used in agriculture to heavy metals like lead and mercury, and even certain food additives—pose significant risks to our health. These substances can enter the body through the food we eat, the water we drink, and even the air we breathe.

Once inside, they can disrupt the delicate balance of the gut microbiome, the community of bacteria and other microorganisms that reside in our digestive system. Research has shown that exposure to these toxins can alter the composition and function of the gut microbiome, leading to an increase in harmful bacteria and a decrease in beneficial ones.

The Impact

The disruption of the gut microbiome by environmental toxins and chemicals can have several detrimental effects on health, including:

- **Increased Inflammation:** Many environmental toxins can trigger an inflammatory response in the gut, which can lead to chronic inflammation, a root cause of many diseases.
- **Impaired Digestion and Absorption:** Toxins can damage the intestinal lining, leading to leaky gut

syndrome, where undigested food particles and toxins leak into the bloodstream, causing further inflammation and immune reactions.
- **Increased Susceptibility to Infections:** A disrupted microbiome can compromise the gut barrier, making it easier for pathogens to enter the body and cause infections.
- **Metabolic Disorders:** There is growing evidence linking environmental toxins to obesity, diabetes, and other metabolic disorders, partly due to their impact on gut microbiota and gut health.

The Solution

Mitigating the impact of environmental toxins on gut health requires a multifaceted approach:

- **Reduce Exposure:** Whenever possible, reduce exposure to known toxins by choosing organic foods, using natural cleaning products, and avoiding areas with high pollution levels. Filtering drinking water can also help remove contaminants.
- **Support Detoxification:** The body's natural detoxification processes can be supported through dietary choices rich in antioxidants and fiber. Foods like leafy greens, berries, garlic, and seeds can boost the body's ability to detoxify harmful substances.
- **Strengthen the Gut Barrier:** Consuming a diet high in prebiotics and probiotics can help maintain a healthy gut microbiome, which supports the integrity

of the gut barrier. Fermented foods like yogurt, kefir, sauerkraut, and kimchi are excellent sources of probiotics, while prebiotic-rich foods include garlic, onions, bananas, and asparagus.
- **Lifestyle Changes:** Regular exercise, adequate sleep, and stress management practices like meditation and yoga can also strengthen the gut barrier and support overall gut health.

By identifying and eliminating environmental gut health disruptors and adopting a lifestyle that supports gut integrity and balance, individuals can take significant steps toward maintaining optimal gut health and overall well-being.

NOURISHING YOUR MICROBIOME: LIFESTYLE CHOICES THAT PROMOTE MICROBIAL DIVERSITY

The health of our gut microbiome extends beyond the realm of diet alone. A variety of lifestyle choices significantly contribute to the rich diversity of our gut microbiota, paving the way for better overall gut health. Here are some key lifestyle elements that can promote and sustain microbial diversity, some of which we briefly touched on in the last chapter.

Regular Exercise

The benefits of regular physical activity extend beyond maintaining physical fitness, it also plays a crucial role in enhancing the diversity of our gut microbiota. Exercise stimulates the growth of various beneficial gut bacteria, which have far-reaching effects on our overall health. Let's dive deeper into this:

The Science

Regular exercise has been shown to increase the diversity of gut bacteria, which is a key indicator of gut health. A diverse microbiome is better equipped to fight off pathogens, break down food, and synthesize essential nutrients and vitamins. Exercise stimulates the growth of beneficial bacteria that produce short-chain fatty acids (SCFAs), such as butyrate, propionate, and acetate. These SCFAs have anti-inflammatory properties, strengthen the gut barrier, and provide energy to our gut cells, thereby promoting a healthy digestive system.

The mechanisms through which exercise affects the gut microbiome are multifaceted and involve several biological pathways:

- **Physical activity increases gut motility**, which can help maintain a healthy balance of gut microbes by preventing the overgrowth of undesirable bacteria.
- **Exercise induces changes in the production of bile acids and other digestive enzymes**, which can influence the composition of the gut microbiome.
- **It also affects the body's stress response**, reducing levels of stress hormones that can negatively impact gut permeability and microbiome composition.
- **Exercise-induced improvements in body composition and metabolic health** can also indirectly benefit gut microbiome diversity and

function, as obesity and metabolic disorders have been linked to less diverse and dysbiotic gut microbial communities.

The Impact

The impact of exercise on the gut microbiome and its subsequent effects on overall health is profound and far-reaching. Regular physical activity can lead to a cascade of positive outcomes across various aspects of health, underlining the interconnectedness of the human body's systems. Here's a summary of the key impacts:

Enhanced Digestive Health

- **Increased Microbial Diversity**: A more diverse gut microbiome, stimulated by regular exercise, improves digestive efficiency and resilience against gastrointestinal disorders.
- **Strengthened Gut Barrier**: Exercise promotes beneficial bacteria that produce short-chain fatty acids, strengthening the gut lining and reducing the risk of leaky gut syndrome.

Improved Immune Function

- **Balanced Immune Response**: A healthy gut microbiome, supported by exercise, plays a crucial role in the development and function of the immune

system, helping to protect against pathogens and reduce inflammation.
- **Lower Infection Rates**: Enhanced immune function can lead to decreased infection susceptibility and possibly faster recovery times.

Mental Health and Cognitive Benefits

- **Mood Regulation**: The production of neurotransmitters by beneficial gut bacteria, encouraged by physical activity, can positively affect mood and reduce the risk of depression and anxiety.
- **Cognitive Function**: There is emerging evidence to suggest that a healthy gut microbiome may influence brain health and cognitive function, potentially lowering the risk of neurodegenerative diseases.

Metabolic and Cardiovascular Health

- **Improved Metabolism**: Regular exercise can lead to alterations in the gut microbiome that enhance metabolic health, reducing the risk of obesity, type 2 diabetes, and metabolic syndrome.
- **Cardiovascular Benefits**: The anti-inflammatory effects of a healthy gut microbiome can contribute to reduced risk of cardiovascular diseases, including hypertension and heart disease.

Longevity and Quality of Life

- **Chronic Disease Prevention**: The cumulative effect of a healthier gut microbiome, due to regular exercise, may contribute to a lower risk of developing chronic diseases, promoting longevity.
- **Enhanced Well-being**: The overall improvement in physical, mental, and emotional health can lead to a better quality of life and well-being.

The Solution

The type and intensity of physical activity can vary based on individual preferences and capabilities, but the key is consistency. Whether it's a brisk walk, a yoga session, or a high-intensity workout, the important thing is to make exercise a part of your daily routine.

So, while we often think of exercise in terms of weight management or cardiovascular health, it's important to remember that regular physical activity also plays a significant role in maintaining a healthy gut. By incorporating some form of exercise into your daily routine, you're not just staying fit, you're also taking a crucial step towards better gut health.

Adequate Sleep

Our sleep-wake cycle, or circadian rhythm, plays a significant role in the health of our gut flora. Disruptions to this cycle, such as irregular sleep patterns or lack of sufficient sleep, can upset the balance of our gut microbiome, potentially leading to various health issues. Let's break this down a bit:

The Science

Our circadian rhythm, which dictates our sleep-wake cycle, has a profound effect on our gut flora. This is because the bacteria in our gut also follow a daily rhythm, with their activities changing between day and night.

The Impact

Disruptions in our sleep-wake cycle can lead to an imbalance in our gut microbiome. This imbalance can pave the way for various health issues, from gastrointestinal problems to weakened immune responses, and even mood disorders.

The Solution

Prioritizing a good night's sleep isn't just about feeling rested—it's a crucial component of gut health. Maintaining a regular sleep schedule and creating a sleep-friendly environment can help promote deep and restorative sleep, which is essential for a balanced gut.

In essence, a good night's sleep is more important than we might think. It is not only vital for our brain function and overall well-being, but it is also crucial for maintaining a healthy gut microbiome. So, don't underestimate the power of a good night's sleep—it's a key part of the puzzle for your gut health.

Hydration

Hydration is a critical factor in maintaining a healthy gut environment. Consuming an adequate amount of fluids, particularly water, not only aids digestion but also maintains the health of our intestines and promotes the efficient removal of waste products. Let's unpack this more:

The Science

Hydration is fundamental to maintaining optimal gut health. Water is essential for various digestive processes, starting from the breakdown of food in the stomach to its eventual absorption in the intestines. Adequate fluid intake ensures that the digestive system functions smoothly, facilitating the breakdown of nutrients for absorption and aiding in the dissolution of soluble fiber, which can help prevent constipation by adding bulk to stools and promoting their movement through the colon.

Moreover, water plays a critical role in maintaining the mucosal lining of the intestines. This lining is vital for nutrient absorption and also acts as a barrier against harmful substances and pathogens. By keeping the mucosal lining well-hydrated, we support its integrity and functionality, thereby enhancing our gut health and overall immune response.

The Impact

The impact of proper hydration on gut health is significant and multifaceted. By ensuring the body is well-hydrated, we support the digestive system in several crucial ways, leading to improved gut health and general well-being. Here are the key impacts:

- **Efficient Digestion and Nutrient Absorption**: Adequate hydration aids in the breakdown of food, allowing the body to absorb nutrients more effectively. Water is essential for dissolving minerals and other nutrients, making them accessible to the body. This efficient nutrient absorption is crucial for energy production, growth, and the maintenance of bodily functions.
- **Prevention of Constipation**: Hydration plays a pivotal role in preventing constipation, a common gastrointestinal issue. Sufficient fluid intake helps to soften stool and promotes its easier passage through the intestines. This not only prevents discomfort but also reduces the risk of complications associated with chronic constipation, such as hemorrhoids and diverticulitis.
- **Maintenance of Intestinal Health**: Water helps to maintain the integrity of the mucosal lining of the intestines, which is vital for protecting the gut from pathogens and facilitating the absorption of nutrients. A well-hydrated mucosal lining supports a healthy balance of gut bacteria, which is essential for digestion, immune function, and even mood regulation.
- **Better Overall Gut Health**: The cumulative effect of efficient digestion, prevention of constipation, and

maintenance of intestinal health leads to better overall gut health. A healthy gut contributes to a stronger immune system, reduces the risk of inflammatory bowel diseases, and supports mental health through the gut-brain axis.

The Solution

Keeping a water bottle handy and making a conscious effort to drink water throughout the day can help ensure that you stay well-hydrated. It's a simple yet effective way to support your gut health.

So, while hydration is often associated with skin health or physical performance, it's also a key component of a healthy gut. By making an effort to stay well-hydrated throughout the day, you're taking a simple but significant step towards better gut health.

Intermittent Fasting

Intermittent fasting (IF) is an eating pattern that cycles between periods of eating and fasting. Typically, this involves abstaining from eating for 16-24 hours at a time. But how can this influence our gut microbiota?

The Science

Intermittent fasting (IF) is an eating pattern that cycles between periods of eating and fasting. Typically, this involves abstaining from eating for 16-24 hours at a time. But how can this influence our gut microbiota?

Scientific studies suggest that intermittent fasting can lead to increased diversity in the gut microbiome, which is an indicator of gut health. Fasting periods appear to provide gut bacteria with a break that allows the microbial community to recover and diversify.

A study published in the journal "Cell Metabolism" showed that IF could alter the gut microbiota in a way that promotes health and longevity. The researchers found that IF influenced the gut microbiota to produce more beneficial metabolites that improve gut health, including butyrate, a short-chain fatty acid that has anti-inflammatory effects and can boost gut barrier function.

The Impact

By increasing microbial diversity and promoting the production of beneficial metabolites, IF can have several positive impacts on gut health. These include improving gut barrier function, reducing inflammation, and potentially decreasing the risk of gut-related diseases.

Moreover, the metabolic changes induced by IF can have broader health benefits. These include improved insulin sensitivity, reduced risk of metabolic syndrome, and potential weight loss (3), making IF a lifestyle choice with both gut-specific and systemic health benefits.

The Solution

Incorporating IF into your lifestyle requires planning and gradual changes. It's essential to choose an IF method that fits your lifestyle, health needs, and dietary preferences. The most common methods include the 16/8 method (fasting for 16 hours and eating within an 8-hour window), the 5:2 diet (eating normally for 5 days and restricting calories for 2 days), or Eat-Stop-Eat (one or two 24-hour fasts per week).

Remember to stay hydrated during fasts, and when you do eat, focus on nutrient-dense foods that support gut health. And, as always, consult with a healthcare professional before starting a new dietary regimen like intermittent fasting.

Mindfulness Practices

Activities that promote mindfulness, such as meditation, yoga, and deep-breathing exercises, are essential tools for managing stress levels. Chronic stress can disrupt our gut microbiome. By participating in mindfulness practices, we can mitigate the effects of stress, promoting a healthier and more balanced gut. Make mindfulness a part of your daily routine—even a few minutes a day can make a significant difference.

Nourishing your gut microbiome involves a comprehensive approach that includes not only a balanced diet but also a healthy lifestyle. By incorporating these elements into your daily routine, you can promote a diverse and robust gut microbiome, leading to better overall health and well-being.

As you continue this journey towards cultivating your inner garden and enhancing your gut health, it's important to remember that the gut is a complex ecosystem. It's not just about the bacteria, but also about the various processes happening within this environment. One such crucial process involves enzymes, the biological catalysts that speed up chemical reactions in our bodies.

These enzymes play a key role in digestion, helping us break down food into nutrients that our bodies can use. In the next chapter, we'll explore the vital role of enzymes in our gut health. We'll delve into how these microscopic powerhouses work, why they're important for our digestion, and how we can support their function for optimal gut health. Stay tuned as we uncover another layer of complexity in our inner garden and reveal ways to give yourself the enzymatic edge.

3
THE ENZYMATIC EDGE

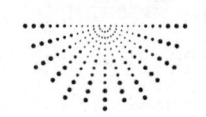

Food indeed plays a pivotal role in our health and well-being. The phrase "Let food be thy medicine, and let medicine be thy food," attributed to Hippocrates, underscores the idea that the quality of the food we consume can impact our overall health.

Hippocrates, often called the "Father of Medicine," was a Greek physician born in 460 BC. His teachings and philosophies, including the Hippocratic Oath - still sworn by doctors today, laid the groundwork for modern Western medicine. He believed in the healing power of nature and asserted that diet, exercise, and rest were critical for maintaining health and treating diseases. This perspective is particularly relevant today, with a growing focus on preventative healthcare and holistic well-being.

Now, back to food as medicine: The food we eat doesn't just satisfy our hunger. It provides the essential nutrients our bodies need to function optimally. These include carbohydrates, proteins, fats, vitamins, and minerals, each playing unique roles in our body's processes like energy production, tissue growth and repair, and immune function.

However, merely consuming nutrient-rich food is not enough. Our bodies must absorb these nutrients effectively for them to be beneficial. Factors such as the health of our digestive system, the way food is prepared, and even the combinations of foods we eat can influence nutrient absorption. For instance, certain vitamins are fat-soluble, meaning they are better absorbed when consumed with dietary fats.

If our bodies are not properly absorbing nutrients, they could just pass through our system without providing their intended benefits. This can lead to nutrient deficiencies, even if we're consuming a seemingly nutritious diet. Paying attention to not only what we eat but also how we eat can help maximize nutrient absorption, allowing food to truly be our medicine.

Understanding the difference between ingestion and absorption is key to optimizing our nutritional intake. Let's unravel this process:

Ingestion vs Absorption

Ingestion is the first step in the digestive process, where food is taken into the body through the mouth. This process involves the act of eating, where food is chewed and mixed with saliva. Saliva contains enzymes that begin the breakdown of carbohydrates. The chewed food then travels down the esophagus and enters the stomach, where it is further broken down by stomach acids and enzymes. However, it's important to note that ingestion merely refers to the intake of food and does not ensure that the nutrients contained in the food are made available to the body.

Absorption: The Key to Nutrient Utilization

After the process of digestion, where food is broken down into its component nutrients, absorption comes into play. This critical phase occurs primarily in the small intestine, where the majority of nutrient absorption takes place. The lining of the small intestine is covered in millions of tiny hair-like structures called villi and microvilli, which significantly increase the surface area for absorption.

As the digested food passes through the small intestine, nutrients such as amino acids (from proteins), fatty acids and glycerol (from fats), vitamins, minerals, and simple sugars (from carbohydrates) are absorbed through the intestinal walls. These nutrients then enter the bloodstream or the lymphatic system, which transports them to various parts of the body where they are utilized for energy, growth, repair, and maintaining bodily functions.

The Importance of Efficient Absorption

The efficiency of nutrient absorption is crucial for the body to benefit from the food consumed. Factors that can affect absorption include the health of the digestive system, the presence of certain digestive enzymes, the bioavailability of nutrients, and interactions between different nutrients. For instance, certain vitamins and minerals are better absorbed in the presence of others, such as vitamin D enhancing calcium absorption.

Inadequate absorption can lead to nutrient deficiencies, even when consuming a nutrient-rich diet. Conditions such as celiac disease, Crohn's disease, and chronic pancreatitis can impair the body's ability to absorb nutrients effectively. Furthermore, lifestyle factors such as excessive alcohol consumption and the use of certain medications can also impact nutrient absorption negatively.

Factors Affecting Absorption

The absorption of nutrients is a complex process influenced by a myriad of factors ranging from the presence of other nutrients and the health of the digestive system to lifestyle factors such as stress levels. Here, we delve into these factors in more detail, supported by real-world studies that highlight the significance of each.

Presence of Other Nutrients

The interaction between different nutrients can significantly affect their absorption. A well-documented example is the relationship between vitamin C and iron. Vitamin C enhances the absorption of non-heme iron (the form of iron found in plant-based foods) by reducing it to a form that is more readily absorbed by the body. A study published in the American Journal of Clinical Nutrition found that consuming 100 mg of vitamin C with a meal increased iron absorption by up to four times.

Similarly, fat-soluble vitamins (A, D, E, and K) require the presence of dietary fat for optimal absorption. A study in the Journal of the Academy of Nutrition and Dietetics showed that adding avocado, a source of healthy fats, to a salad increased the absorption of alpha-carotene, beta-carotene, and lutein, which are nutrients important for eye health and immune function.

Gut Health

The health of the gastrointestinal tract plays a crucial role in nutrient absorption. Conditions such as celiac disease, inflammatory bowel disease (IBD), and irritable bowel syndrome (IBS) can impair the absorption of nutrients by damaging the lining of the gut or causing inflammation. A review in the World Journal of Gastroenterology highlights that individuals with celiac disease often suffer from deficiencies in iron, calcium, and B vitamins due to malabsorption.

The gut microbiota, the complex community of microorganisms living in the digestive tract, also influences nutrient absorption. Probiotics, beneficial bacteria that can be consumed through certain foods or supplements, have been shown to improve the absorption of minerals such as calcium, iron, and zinc, as demonstrated in a meta-analysis published in Nutrients.

Stress Levels

Chronic stress can negatively impact gut health and, consequently, nutrient absorption. Stress affects the gut-brain axis, leading to changes in gastrointestinal motility, an increase in intestinal permeability (sometimes referred to as "leaky gut"), and alterations in the gut microbiota. These changes can impair the body's ability to absorb nutrients. A study in the journal Gut Microbes discusses how stress-induced alterations in the gut microbiota can affect the absorption of nutrients, highlighting the importance of managing stress for optimal digestive health.

Real-World Implications

Understanding the factors affecting nutrient absorption can inform dietary choices and lifestyle changes to improve health outcomes. For example, individuals can enhance iron absorption by consuming vitamin C-rich foods alongside iron-rich meals, especially if they are vegetarian or vegan and rely on non-heme iron sources. Incorporating healthy fats into meals can improve the absorption of fat-soluble vitamins, supporting overall health.

Moreover, addressing gut health issues through diet, probiotics, and stress management can improve nutrient absorption and prevent deficiencies. These strategies underscore the interconnectedness of diet, lifestyle, and health, highlighting the importance of a holistic approach to nutrition and well-being.

Enhancing Nutrient Absorption

Certain practices can enhance nutrient absorption. Consuming a balanced diet rich in a variety of foods can ensure you get a mix of nutrients that support each other's absorption. Hydration, regular exercise, and managing stress also play a vital role in optimizing absorption and we will discuss these in more detail in the next chapter.

As another renowned saying by Ann Wigmore goes, "The food you eat can be either the safest and most powerful form of medicine or the slowest form of poison". So, it's not just about what you eat, but how your body processes what you eat. By understanding and improving nutrient absorption, we can truly let food be our medicine.

THE ROLE OF ENZYMES IN DIGESTION: HOW ENZYMES WORK TO BREAK DOWN FOOD

Enzymes play a crucial role in our digestion. They're like the machinery in a factory, breaking down the food we eat into smaller, manageable parts that our body can use. This isn't a one-size-fits-all process, though. Different enzymes are specialized to break down different types of nutrients.

Proteases break down proteins into amino acids. Lipases break down fats into fatty acids and glycerol. Carbohydrases, like amylase and sucrase, break down complex carbohydrates into simple sugars. Each of these enzymes has a specific pH and temperature at which they work best, creating a complex system of checks and balances to ensure optimal digestion.

Now, let's look at some real-world studies that have enhanced our understanding of these enzymes.

A study published in the Journal of Biological Chemistry in 2011, titled "Function and Structure of a Prokaryotic Formylglycine Amidohydrolase," discovered a new enzyme in our digestive system. This enzyme, called Rhodococcus jostii, helps break down complex carbohydrates, contributing to our understanding of how our bodies process these types of foods.

A 2012 study published in Nature, titled "Gut Microbiota Metabolism of Dietary Fiber Influences Allergic Airway Disease and Hematopoiesis," demonstrated the role of enzymes produced by gut bacteria in breaking down dietary fiber. The researchers found that a diet high in fiber led to a more diverse gut microbiota, with the bacteria producing more enzymes to break down the fiber. This, in turn, resulted in a healthier immune response.

Another study, from the Journal of Lipid Research in 2010, titled "Pancreatic Lipase and Lipase-Related Protein 2, But Not Lipase-Related Protein 1, Hydrolyze Retinyl Palmitate in Physiological Conditions," explored the role of lipases in fat digestion. Through their research, they found that certain lipases were more effective at breaking down specific types of fats, deepening our understanding of fat digestion and absorption.

These studies underscore the crucial role of enzymes in our digestive process. Understanding how these enzymes function can help us better manage our diet and overall health, giving us the power to support our digestive system and, by extension, our overall well-being.

IDENTIFYING ENZYME INSUFFICIENCY: SYMPTOMS AND SOLUTIONS

Enzyme insufficiency is a condition in which your body doesn't produce enough enzymes to ensure proper digestion. This can lead to a variety of uncomfortable symptoms and can affect overall health.

Symptoms

Enzyme insufficiency, also known as enzyme deficiency, is a health condition where your body doesn't produce enough digestive enzymes to properly break down and absorb food. This can result in a range of symptoms, reflecting the body's struggle to optimally digest and utilize nutrients. Let's delve a bit further into these:

- **Bloating and Gas**: Digestive enzymes help break down complex food particles into simpler substances that the body can use. When these enzymes are insufficient, food isn't broken down as it should be, leading it to ferment in the gut and produce gas. This causes uncomfortable bloating and flatulence.
- **Stomach Pain**: Undigested food particles can irritate the lining of the stomach and intestines. This irritation can result in stomach pain or discomfort, often experienced as cramping, aching, or a sense of fullness.
- **Diarrhea or Constipation**: Both of these conditions can result from improper food digestion. Undigested

food can speed up or slow down the transit time of waste through your intestines, resulting in diarrhea or constipation, respectively.
- **Fatigue**: If your body is not properly digesting and absorbing nutrients due to enzyme insufficiency, it can lead to malnutrition over time. Lack of essential nutrients can cause fatigue, as your body isn't getting the energy it needs to function effectively.

These symptoms can significantly impact a person's quality of life. If you or someone else is experiencing these symptoms consistently, it's important to seek medical advice. Treatments may involve dietary changes or enzyme supplementation under the guidance of a healthcare professional.

Solutions

Managing enzyme insufficiency generally requires a two-pronged approach: dietary adjustments and enzyme supplementation. Here's a more detailed look at both:

- **Dietary Adjustments**: Consuming a diet abundant in raw fruits and vegetables can greatly benefit individuals with enzyme insufficiency. These foods naturally contain digestive enzymes that can aid in the breakdown and absorption of nutrients. For instance, pineapples have bromelain and papayas contain papain, both of which aid in protein digestion. However, it's crucial to note that these enzymes are often destroyed by cooking, hence the

emphasis on raw consumption. Additionally, a balanced diet that's high in fiber can also support overall digestive health. Fiber adds bulk to the diet, aids in moving food through the digestive tract, and supports a healthy gut microbiome, which plays a role in digestion and nutrient absorption.
- **Enzyme Supplements**: These are products designed to directly increase enzyme levels in the body. They typically contain a mixture of various enzymes, such as proteases for protein digestion, lipases for fat digestion, and amylases for carbohydrate digestion.

Enzyme supplements can be particularly beneficial for people with conditions like pancreatitis, cystic fibrosis, or any disease that impairs the body's ability to produce or release digestive enzymes. These supplements work by supplying the enzymes that the body is unable to produce on its own, aiding in the digestion process and alleviating digestive discomfort.

Remember, while these solutions can help manage enzyme insufficiency, it's always best to consult with a healthcare provider before making any significant dietary changes or starting a new supplement regimen. They can provide personalized advice based on the individual's health history and current condition.

Always consult a healthcare provider to diagnose enzyme insufficiency and determine the best course of action.

Understanding enzyme insufficiency and its symptoms is the first step in managing this condition. By making appropriate dietary changes and considering enzyme supplements, you can support your body's digestion and overall health.

ENHANCING YOUR ENZYMATIC ACTIVITY: FOODS AND HABITS THAT BOOST YOUR ENZYME POWER

First, let's clarify what enzymes are. Enzymes are proteins that accelerate various biochemical reactions in our bodies, playing a fundamental role in digestion, metabolism, and other essential bodily functions. But, like every other element in our bodies, the production and activity of these enzymes can be influenced by our diet and lifestyle.

Foods that Boost Enzyme Production

Eating certain foods can naturally increase your body's enzyme production. These are mainly raw fruits and vegetables, as cooking can often destroy the enzymes present in these foods.

Foods that Enhance Enzymatic Activity

- **Fermented Foods**: Fermented foods such as yogurt, kefir, sauerkraut, and kimchi are rich in probiotics, which can enhance the body's production of digestive enzymes. These beneficial bacteria contribute to the breakdown of food substances, aiding in their digestion and absorption. Research published in the *Journal of Applied Microbiology* highlights the positive impact of fermented foods on digestive health, attributing it to the enzymatic activity of probiotics.
- **Pineapple and Papaya**: Pineapple contains bromelain, and papaya contains papain, both of which are proteolytic enzymes that help break down

proteins into amino acids. Including these fruits in your diet can aid digestion, particularly of protein-rich foods. A study in the *Biomedical Reports* journal discusses the therapeutic potential of bromelain in treating gastrointestinal disorders due to its enzymatic action.

- **Honey**: Raw honey is another source of natural enzymes, including amylase (which breaks down carbohydrates) and protease (which breaks down proteins). Consuming raw honey, especially when added to warm (not hot) foods or drinks, can introduce these enzymes into the digestive system, supporting the breakdown and absorption of nutrients.

- **Sprouted Seeds, Grains, and Legumes**: Sprouting increases the enzyme content of seeds, grains, and legumes, making them easier to digest. The sprouting process activates food enzymes, improves nutrient bioavailability, and reduces antinutrients, which can inhibit enzyme function. A publication in the *Journal of Nutritional Science and Vitaminology* found that sprouted grains have higher enzyme activity, which can benefit digestive health.

Imagine a vibrant, colorful chart here showcasing these foods with their associated enzymes.

Habits to Enhance Enzyme Activity

Throughout this guide, you will encounter repeated references to specific habits and dietary choices that are essential for enhancing enzymatic activity and, more broadly, for protecting and nurturing our gut health. This repetition is intentional and serves a crucial purpose: to lock in the importance of these practices in maintaining and improving digestive health, which is foundational to overall well-being. Here are a few tips for enhancing your enzyme activity:

Habits that Boost Enzyme Power

Hydration: Adequate hydration is essential for enzymatic activity. Enzymes require a certain amount of water to function optimally. Drinking sufficient water throughout the day can ensure that all biochemical reactions, including those catalyzed by enzymes, proceed efficiently.

Eating Mindful: Chewing food thoroughly is crucial for enzyme function. Saliva contains digestive enzymes such as amylase and lipase, which begin the digestive process in the mouth. By chewing food well, you maximize the contact time with these enzymes, improving the breakdown of nutrients.

Managing Stress: Chronic stress can negatively impact enzyme production and secretion, particularly those involved in digestion. Stress management techniques, such as mindfulness, yoga, and regular physical activity, can help maintain optimal enzymatic activity by reducing the adverse effects of stress on the body.

Regular Exercise: Physical activity can boost overall enzyme function by enhancing blood circulation, which ensures that enzymes and nutrients are efficiently transported throughout the body. Regular exercise also supports the health of the digestive system, further improving nutrient breakdown and absorption.

Envision a diagram here indicating the correlation between these lifestyle habits and enzyme production.

By consciously choosing enzyme-rich foods and adopting healthy habits, you can naturally enhance your enzymatic activity. This will not only optimize your digestion but also contribute to your overall well-being. Remember, every small step towards a healthier lifestyle counts. Here's to boosting your enzyme power!

As we've explored, harnessing the power of enzymes is a catalyst for improved health and well-being. By integrating enzyme-rich foods and adopting enzymatically supportive habits, we've set the stage for a healthier, more vibrant life. But there's more to health than impressive enzymatic activity. Now, we're going to shift gears and delve into another crucial aspect of our health – the immune system.

Just as a well-oiled machine relies on its components to function optimally, our bodies depend on a robust immune system to ward off disease and maintain health. In the following chapter, we will explore how to strengthen this intricate defense network, turning it into an impregnable fortress. From nutrient-packed foods to beneficial lifestyle changes, let's continue our journey toward optimal health.

4
FORTIFYING YOUR IMMUNE FORTRESS

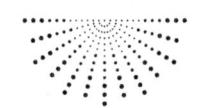

Did you know that a staggering 70% of your immune system is housed right in your gut? I hope so as it was touched on in chapter 1 but yes, it's true! This surprising fact reveals the profound link between gut health and immune function. So when you hear health enthusiasts talking about 'gut flora' and 'microbiome', it's no fad. As we journey further, we're going to delve into the complex ties between your gut health and your body's defense mechanisms.

Let us explore how nurturing your gut's billions of residents can be a secret weapon in amplifying your immunity. So buckle up and get ready to dive into this captivating world where gut health intersects with immune function. We're on a mission to unlock the door to peak health and vitality.

THE IMMUNE SYSTEM'S COMMAND CENTER: THE GUT'S ROLE IN IMMUNITY

The gut, commonly perceived as merely a component of our digestive system, is a core element of our immune system. It is a bustling ecosystem teeming with trillions of microbes that collectively form our gut microbiota. These diverse microbes are not just passive residents, they are active contributors to our well-being, playing an instrumental role in reinforcing our immune defenses.

Recent years have seen a surge in scientific interest in the link between the gut and our immune system. This curiosity stems from the growing realization that our gut microbiota exerts a profound influence on our immunity. Surprisingly, the gut is the site where our body's immune cells mature and learn their functions. This is where our immune system learns the intricate dance of distinguishing between harmful pathogens and benign entities, such as food particles and beneficial bacteria.

The human gut, often viewed as a simple organ for digestion, is a complex ecosystem and a pivotal component of our immune system. The gut-associated lymphoid tissue (GALT) is a key player in this context. GALT is like the immune system's classroom, where over 70% of our immune cells learn and mature.

These immune cells undergo a process of education in the gut, learning to differentiate between harmful pathogens, such as disease-causing bacteria or viruses, and benign entities like food particles and beneficial bacteria. Just like students in a classroom, these cells need to learn the difference between friends (beneficial bacteria and food particles) and foes (harmful pathogens) to respond appropriately.

The Role of Microbiota in Immune System Maturation

The interaction between the gut microbiota and the immune system is a sophisticated dialogue that influences the immune cells' development and function. These microbes engage in constant communication with immune cells, guiding their responses to various antigens and teaching them to differentiate between harmful invaders and harmless entities. This microbial "education" of the immune system is fundamental to its ability to protect the body against pathogens while preventing autoimmune responses.

Regulatory T Cells (Tregs) and Immune Tolerance

A key aspect of this microbial teaching process involves the stimulation of regulatory T cells (Tregs) by certain beneficial gut bacteria. Tregs are a subset of T cells that play an indispensable role in maintaining immune tolerance. They help the immune system avoid overreacting to non-harmful antigens, such as food particles or commensal bacteria, and prevent it from attacking the body's own tissues. The production and function of Tregs are significantly influenced by signals from gut microbes, highlighting the gut microbiota's critical role in developing and maintaining immune tolerance.

Mechanisms of Microbial Influence on the Immune System

The mechanisms through which the gut microbiota influences immune system maturation are diverse and complex. These include:

- **Metabolic Products:** Microbial metabolites, such as short-chain fatty acids (SCFAs), produced through the fermentation of dietary fibers, can modulate immune cell behavior, promoting the development of Tregs and enhancing the gut barrier function.
- **Microbial Antigens:** Exposure to a wide variety of microbial antigens in the gut helps to train the immune system, improving its ability to recognize and respond to pathogens while tolerating non-pathogenic antigens.
- **Direct Cellular Interactions:** Some gut bacteria can directly interact with the cells of the gut lining and immune cells, facilitating the development of oral tolerance and the maturation of immune responses.

The Immune System's Dance: Recognizing Friend and Foe

In the complex world of human biology, the immune system performs an intricate ballet, constantly distinguishing between friend and foe. This sophisticated system safeguards our health by identifying and neutralizing harmful pathogens while simultaneously preserving a harmonious relationship with beneficial microbes and the body's cells. Understanding the mechanisms underlying this delicate balance provides insights into immune function, potential vulnerabilities, and the pathways to enhancing disease resistance.

The Cast of the Immune Dance

At the heart of this performance are the immune cells, the dancers in this metaphorical ballet. These cells circulate throughout the body, vigilantly scanning for signs of infection or disease. Key players include T cells, B cells, macrophages, dendritic cells, and natural killer cells, each with specific roles in defense and tolerance.

- **T cells**, especially regulatory T cells (Tregs), are akin to choreographers, directing the immune response to maintain tolerance to self-antigens and benign environmental substances.
- **B cells** produce antibodies, tagging pathogens for destruction or neutralization—a performance that memorizes and targets specific threats.
- **Macrophages and dendritic cells** act as scouts, engulfing pathogens and presenting their antigens to T cells, initiating a targeted immune response.
- **Natural killer cells** patrol the body, ready to eliminate cells that have become infected or transformed into cancer cells.

The immune system's ability to recognize friend from foe hinges on a complex network of signals and checkpoints. Antigen presentation and the subsequent activation or suppression of immune cells are critical steps in this process. The system's specificity and memory allow it to swiftly respond to previously encountered pathogens while remaining adaptable to new threats.

Challenges in the Immune Dance

Disruptions in the immune system's ability to distinguish between harmful and harmless can lead to autoimmune diseases, allergies, and chronic inflammatory conditions. Factors contributing to these disruptions include genetic predispositions, environmental triggers, and changes in the gut microbiota.

Strategies to enhance the immune system's function and ensure its correct recognition of friend and foe are areas of active research and intervention. These include:

- **Nutritional support:** to nourish the gut microbiota and immune cells.
- **Immunotherapy:** for allergies and autoimmune diseases, recalibrating the immune response towards tolerance.
- **Probiotics and prebiotics:** to support a healthy gut microbiota, influencing immune system education and function.

The Impact of Lifestyle Choices on Gut Microbiota and Immunity

Our lifestyle choices, such as diet, exercise, sleep, and stress management, can significantly influence the composition and diversity of our gut microbiota, which in turn impacts our immune system's function and overall health. For instance, a diet rich in diverse plant-based foods can promote a diverse gut microbiota, which is associated with a strong and balanced immune response.

Here's a table to summarize the effects of different lifestyle factors on gut microbiota and immunity:

Lifestyle Factor	Impact on Gut Microbiota	Impact on Immunity
Diet	Diverse, fiber-rich diets promote a diverse and balanced gut microbiota.	A balanced gut microbiota supports a strong and balanced immune response.
Exercise	Regular exercise can enhance gut microbial diversity.	Exercise can boost immune function and reduce inflammation.
Sleep	Disrupted sleep can alter gut microbiota composition.	Poor sleep can impair immune function.
Stress	Chronic stress can disrupt gut microbial balance.	Stress can weaken immune responses and increase susceptibility to infection.

Groundbreaking research by Thaiss et al. (2016) showed for the first time that the gut microbiota can influence the circadian rhythm of the host's immune system. In simpler terms, our gut bacteria can instruct our immune system when to ramp up or dial down its activity, effectively acting as a timekeeper for our immunity. This finding underscores the gut's pivotal role as the command center for the immune system.

Further, a 2018 study published in the journal 'Nature' showed that the gut microbiota influences how immune cells develop and function, shaping the body's immunity at a fundamental level. When there is an imbalance in the gut microbiota, known as dysbiosis, it can lead to a weakened immune system and increased susceptibility to infections and diseases.

Yet, there's more. A 2020 study in 'Cell' discovered that the gut microbiota can also stimulate the production of a type of immune cell called Th17 cells. These cells are responsible for maintaining the integrity of the gut lining and protecting against harmful pathogens. This study showcases another mechanism through which the gut microbiota bolsters our immunity.

In light of these findings, it's clear that the gut is far from just a digestive organ. It's a vital part of our immune system and a central hub where important decisions about our immunity are made. The gut microbiota, with its myriad microbes, plays the role of an ally, collaborator, and guide in this process, shaping our immune responses in ways we are only just beginning to understand.

ALLIES IN IMMUNITY: PROBIOTICS AND THEIR CONTRIBUTION TO YOUR DEFENSE SYSTEM

Probiotics, often called 'good bacteria', are live microorganisms that can provide health benefits when consumed in sufficient amounts. They are a critical part of our gut microbiota and play a pivotal role in our immune system functionality.

Several mechanisms are at play in how probiotics contribute to our immune health. Not only do they compete with harmful bacteria for nutrients and attachment sites in the gut, thereby maintaining a healthy balance, but they also stimulate the production of natural antibodies. Furthermore, they boost the function of immune cells such as T lymphocytes and Natural Killer cells, key players in our body's defense system.

A thorough review by Plaza-Díaz et al. in 2017 demonstrated that different strains of probiotics could effectively modulate the immune response, potentially preventing the onset of immune and inflammatory disorders. This research highlights the significant impact these tiny gut inhabitants can have on our immune health.

Furthering this topic, a study by West et al. (2014) found that a certain strain of Lactobacillus rhamnosus could reduce the incidence of respiratory infections in children. Similarly, research by King et al. (2014) showed that supplementation with Bifidobacterium Animalis Subsp. Lactis reduces the incidence of acute respiratory tract infections in healthy physically active individuals.

A meta-analysis conducted by Hao et al. (2015) found that probiotic consumption significantly improved the general health status of elderly people by enhancing their immune function, demonstrating the beneficial effects of probiotics on a demographic that often faces immune decline.

Probiotics are live microorganisms that, when consumed in adequate amounts, confer health benefits to the host, primarily by supporting a healthy gut microbiome. Different strains of probiotics offer somewhat different benefits, but overall, they contribute to a healthy digestive system and may boost the immune system. Here's a deeper dive into some probiotics.

Lactobacillus

This is a common type of bacteria found in the gut and in certain fermented foods. Different strains, such as Lactobacillus rhamnosus and Lactobacillus Acidophilus, have been studied for their health benefits. These strains are known to support gut health by inhibiting harmful bacteria, improving the gut barrier function, and promoting the healthy balance of gut flora. Moreover, they have been linked with enhanced immunity by stimulating the body's natural defense mechanisms.

Bifidobacterium

These bacteria are part of the natural gut microbiota and can be found in various types of fermented foods. Strains like Bifidobacterium Longum and Bifidobacterium Bifidum have been associated with improved gut health and enhanced immunity. They function by inhibiting harmful bacteria, promoting a balanced gut environment, and stimulating the immune response.

Saccharomyces boulardii

Unlike the others, this is a probiotic yeast. It's been linked with improved gut health and enhanced immune function. It's particularly known for its efficacy against diarrhea, including that caused by antibiotics or travel.

Super Probiotics

Some probiotics, due to their extensive health benefits and robust scientific backing, are often referred to as 'super probiotics'. Examples include Lactobacillus Casei Shirota and Bifidobacterium Lactis Bb12. They've been associated with a wide range of benefits, from improved gut health and immunity to potential benefits for mental health and weight management.

While probiotics can support immune health and promote a healthy gut, they're not a magic bullet. They should be used as part of an overall healthy lifestyle, including a balanced diet and regular exercise. As always, it's crucial to consult with a healthcare professional before starting a new supplement regimen to ensure it's suitable for your unique health needs.

Lactobacillus Casei Shirota

This probiotic strain is well known for its extensive health benefits, especially in terms of gut health and immunity. It's been associated with improved digestion, reduced risk of antibiotic-associated diarrhea, and even potential benefits for mental health. You can find this strain in fermented dairy products like yogurt and cheese. One of the most common sources is a probiotic drink called Yakult, which was specifically developed with this strain.

Bifidobacterium Lactis Bb12

Bifidobacterium Lactis Bb12 is another 'super probiotic' that comes with a range of health benefits. It's been linked to improved digestion, enhanced immune function, and even potential benefits for weight management. This strain is often found in fermented foods like yogurt, kefir, and sauerkraut. Certain probiotic supplements also contain this strain.

Remember that while these super probiotics can support gut health and immunity, they are not a panacea. They work best when incorporated into a healthy lifestyle that includes a balanced diet and regular exercise. Also, it's crucial to consult with a healthcare professional before starting any new supplement regimen, as what works best will depend on your health circumstances and needs.

Lastly, it's important to note that the quality of probiotic products can vary widely. Make sure to choose products from reputable brands that guarantee the potency of their products until the end of their shelf life.

LIFESTYLE IMMUNE BOOSTERS: DAILY PRACTICES TO STRENGTHEN YOUR IMMUNE RESPONSE

While the gut plays a significant role in our immune system, it doesn't work in isolation. Our lifestyle choices also have a direct impact on our immune health. Good nutrition, regular exercise, adequate sleep, and stress management are some of the key lifestyle factors that can help boost our immune system.

Fortifying our immune system is a multi-faceted process. By understanding the crucial role our gut plays, harnessing the power of probiotics, and adopting a healthy lifestyle, we can build a robust immune system that's ready to protect us from whatever comes our way.

nurturing our gut health is not just about aiding digestion—it's about creating a thriving ecosystem that can support our immunity. As we've seen, the gut is the command center of our immune system, and probiotics are some of our most powerful allies in this fight. Therefore, adopting a lifestyle that supports this intricate gut-immune connection is essential for overall health.

Practice	Benefits	Details
Diet	Fuels immune function	Eat fruits, vegetables, lean proteins, healthy fats. They're rich in supporting vitamins, minerals, antioxidants.
Exercise	Boosts circulation	Regular activities like jogging, swimming, walking improve circulation, reduce inflammation.
Sleep	Regulates immunity	Aim for 7-9 hours. Sleep helps produce cytokines, proteins targeting infection, inflammation.
Stress Management	Enhances immune health	Try yoga, meditation, mindfulness. Reducing stress prevents hormonal imbalances suppressing immunity.

Balanced Diet

A balanced diet is indeed our first line of defense, but daily life can often make it difficult to maintain. Between work, school, or family responsibilities, finding time to prepare nutritious meals can be a struggle. Fast food or processed meals may seem like time-saving alternatives, but they often lack the essential nutrients our immune system requires.

Micronutrients such as vitamins and minerals are critical for immune responses. However, it's worth noting that these nutrients are most beneficial when obtained from whole foods, rather than supplements. The body absorbs these nutrients more efficiently from food, and whole foods also provide a complex mix of beneficial compounds.

Consistency is key here. Even small steps towards a healthier diet, like adding more fruits and vegetables to your meals, or swapping processed snacks for whole foods, can make a big difference over time. Remember, a balanced diet isn't about perfection but about making healthier choices more often.

Regular Exercise

Regular, moderate exercise can enhance immune function. However, our daily routines can often make it challenging to find time to exercise. Long working hours, family commitments, or even a lack of motivation can be significant hurdles.

It's important to remember that exercise doesn't necessarily mean spending hours at the gym. It can be as simple as taking a brisk walk during your lunch break, doing a quick workout at home, or even taking the stairs instead of the elevator. The key is to be consistent and to find an activity you enjoy, which will make it easier to stick with it long-term.

Exercise promotes good circulation, allowing immune cells to move freely and work more efficiently. And while it's crucial to be consistent with exercise, it's equally important not to overdo it. Intense, prolonged exercise without sufficient recovery can suppress the immune system, so balance is essential.

Sleep

Sleep is a vital aspect of our overall health, including our immune function. However, the demands and distractions of daily life can often disrupt our sleep patterns. Stress from work or personal issues, the allure of late-night entertainment or social media, or even the lack of a regular sleep schedule can all lead to insufficient sleep.

The impact of sleep on our immune system is significant. As per the study by Besedovsky et al., 2019, sleep and our body's circadian system have a strong influence on immune functions.

When our sleep is disrupted or insufficient, it can weaken our immune system and make us more susceptible to infections.

Now, think about how often we compromise our sleep due to the demands of daily life. Maybe we stay up late to finish a work project, or we sacrifice sleep to binge-watch a favorite show. These inconsistent sleep patterns can be detrimental to our immune health in the long run.

Consistency, once again, is the key. It's crucial to establish a regular sleep schedule and stick to it, even on weekends. Avoiding screens close to bedtime, creating a restful environment, and incorporating a relaxing pre-sleep routine can all contribute to better sleep quality.

Furthermore, it's not just about the quantity of sleep, quality matters too. Deep, restful sleep stages are when the body performs a lot of its repair work, including bolstering the immune system. So, ensuring you get quality sleep is just as important as getting enough hours.

Despite the challenges of daily life, prioritizing and maintaining consistent sleep habits can significantly improve the strength of our immune system over time. It's another instance where small, consistent changes can lead to substantial long-term benefits.

Stress Management

Navigating through life's daily demands and challenges can sometimes be stressful. Whether it's work-related pressure, financial worries, or personal concerns, stress is a common part of our lives. However, how we manage this stress can significantly impact our immune health.

Chronic stress can suppress our immune response, making us more susceptible to infections and illnesses. According to a study by Dhabhar, 2014, stress can dysregulate immune function, adding another layer of importance to stress management.

However, managing stress amid a busy life can be a challenge. We often push aside our mental health needs to meet our daily responsibilities. However, consistently high levels of stress without effective coping mechanisms can take a toll on our immune health.

That's where stress management techniques come into play. They can help us regulate our stress levels and boost our immune system. Here are a few effective stress management techniques:

- **Mindfulness and Meditation:** These practices can help us stay present and focused, reducing our stress levels.
- **Exercise:** Regular physical activity can lower stress levels and improve mood by releasing endorphins, the body's natural stress-relievers.
- **Healthy Eating:** A balanced diet can help manage stress levels. Certain foods can even reduce stress, such as those rich in omega-3 fatty acids and vitamin C.
- **Deep Breathing:** Deep, slow breaths can help relax and reduce tension.
- **Yoga and Tai Chi:** These activities combine physical movement with mindfulness and deep breathing, providing a comprehensive stress management approach.

- **Adequate Sleep:** Quality sleep can help regulate your mood and decrease stress levels.
- **Social Connections:** Spending time with loved ones or speaking to a trusted friend or family member can help reduce feelings of stress.
- **Time Management:** Good time management can help prevent situations that cause stress.
- **Hobbies:** Engaging in activities you enjoy is a great way to reduce stress as they can provide a sense of accomplishment and satisfaction.

Managing stress effectively is crucial for maintaining a robust immune system. Despite the pressures of daily life, incorporating consistent and effective stress management techniques can help bolster our immune health.

Nurturing our immune system is a multi-faceted process. By understanding the crucial role our gut plays, harnessing the power of super probiotics, and adopting healthy lifestyle practices, we can fortify our immune system. It's about creating a thriving ecosystem that supports our immunity, making it ready to protect us from whatever comes our way.

Now that we've understood the crucial role of the gut in our immune system and the importance of a healthy lifestyle, it's time to turn our attention to the next vital step: Purifying Your Gut. The journey towards optimal health always begins from within. The following chapter will delve into the various ways to purify and cleanse our gut, ensuring a healthier and happier you. Stay tuned as we uncover the secrets to a detoxified and well-functioning gut.

5
PURIFYING YOUR GUT

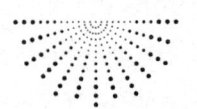

It's rather mind-boggling to think that your gut, often overlooked in the grand scheme of your body's functions, is a bustling metropolis of over 100 trillion bacteria, outnumbering human cells 10 to 1. This diverse collective, known as the gut microbiome, is not just a passive resident. It plays a crucial role in a myriad of functions, from aiding digestion to regulating your immune system, and even influencing your mood. Perhaps most fascinating of all is its significant role in the detoxification process, the body's natural way of purifying itself from harmful substances.

Here's something you might find intriguing about the detox process, it's not just the harmful substances we ingest that need to be detoxified. Our bodies naturally produce waste products from regular metabolic processes that must also be eliminated. Urea, a byproduct of protein metabolism, and bilirubin, a waste product from the breakdown of red blood cells, are two key examples of substances that your detox systems handle daily.

So, in essence, detoxification is a continuous process that's crucial for our survival, not just something we need after overindulging during the holidays.

THE DETOXIFICATION PATHWAYS IN YOUR GUT: HOW YOUR BODY NATURALLY DETOXIFIES

Our bodies are continuously exposed to a myriad of toxins, from the food we eat and the air we breathe to the products we use every day. While this may seem daunting, the human body is remarkably equipped to handle this onslaught. It possesses a complex and intricate detoxification system designed to protect us from damage and maintain our health.

At the forefront of this detoxification system is the gut, an often overlooked yet crucial organ in this process. The gut is much more than just a digestive system component, it's a dynamic ecosystem bustling with trillions of bacteria collectively known as the gut microbiota. These microbes, each playing a different role, work in tandem with the liver, the body's primary detox organ, to efficiently eliminate harmful substances.

The liver and gut microbiota's collaboration is akin to a well-orchestrated symphony, with each component performing its part to maintain the body's harmony. The liver initiates the detoxification process by filtering the blood and breaking down the toxins into less harmful substances. These substances are then further processed by the gut microbiota, which neutralizes them and facilitates their elimination from the body.

However, this detoxification process is not invincible. Factors such as poor diet, stress, lack of sleep, or overuse of antibiotics can disrupt the gut microbiota's balance, leading to a condition known as dysbiosis. Dysbiosis can impair the gut's detoxification abilities, underscoring the importance of maintaining a healthy and balanced gut microbiome.

This chapter will take you on a deep dive into the fascinating world of gut detoxification. We'll explore the liver's role, the gut microbiota's various functions, and the impact of dysbiosis on our body's detoxification. By understanding these processes, we can better appreciate the gut's crucial role in our health and well-being and learn how to nurture this essential organ.

The Role of the Liver in Detoxification

When we think of detoxification, the liver often takes center stage, and for good reason. This vital organ serves as the body's primary processing center for toxins, ensuring they're rendered harmless and efficiently eliminated. It's a two-step dance, involving Phase I and Phase II detoxification, both of which have distinct but interconnected roles.

Phase I Detoxification

Often referred to as the 'activation phase,' this is the initial step in the liver's detoxification process. This phase is predominantly about preparation. It's like the opening act of a play, setting the stage for what's to come.

During Phase I, the liver uses enzymes, specifically a group known as Cytochrome P450, to start breaking down toxins. This family of enzymes is quite versatile, and capable of handling a wide range of substances. These could be environmental pollutants we breathe in, drugs we consume, alcohol we drink, or even waste products from our own bodies' metabolic processes.

The goal of this phase is to transform these toxins into less harmful substances, making them easier for the body to handle and eliminate. Think of it as breaking down a large, unwieldy rock into smaller pieces that are easier to manage.

However, there's a flip side to this. The byproducts of the breakdown process can sometimes be more harmful and reactive than the original toxins. It's akin to the smaller pieces of rock being sharper and more dangerous if not handled correctly.

Phase II Detoxification

This stage of the process, also known as the 'conjugation phase,' is where the liver steps in to neutralize these potentially harmful byproducts from Phase I. If Phase I is the opening act, think of Phase II as the main event where the real action happens.

During Phase II, the liver attaches various molecules to these byproducts, a process known as conjugation. This process transforms these metabolites into water-soluble compounds. Why is this important? Well, by making them water-soluble, the liver is essentially packaging these toxins for easier elimination from the body, mainly through urine and bile.

Phase II is like a sophisticated disposal system, ensuring these toxins are safely and effectively removed from the body with minimal damage.

However, it's crucial to note that the two phases need to work in harmony. If Phase I is working overtime, or Phase II isn't up to speed, it could result in a harmful build-up of toxic metabolites. This underlines the importance of maintaining a healthy liver for an effective detoxification process.

The Role of the Gut Microbiota in Detoxification

The gut microbiota, an incredibly diverse community of microbes that call our intestines home, is essentially an unsung hero when it comes to detoxification. Housing trillions of bacteria, yeasts, and viruses, this microbiome plays a crucial role in maintaining our health, not least in the field of detoxification.

But how exactly does this bustling microbial city help detoxify our bodies? Here are three key ways:

Metabolizing Toxins Directly

Some of the residents of our gut microbiota are incredibly efficient at breaking down toxins directly, acting a bit like the body's own waste disposal unit. For example, research by Li et al. (2018) highlighted the detoxifying power of Lactobacillus bacteria. The study found that certain strains of these bacteria could metabolize and detoxify aflatoxin B1, which is a potent carcinogen. It's like having a resident superhero in your gut, battling villains on a microscopic scale.

Modifying Bile Acids

Bile acids are a bit like the liver's own detergent, helping to digest fats and remove waste from the body. However, some gut bacteria have the unique ability to modify these bile acids, transforming them into secondary bile acids. This transformation aids in the detoxification process, providing an extra layer of assistance to the liver's activities. It's akin to an upgrade, taking a useful tool and making it even more effective in its job.

Producing Short-Chain Fatty Acids (SCFAs)

Certain microbes in our gut are excellent at producing SCFAs, such as butyrate, propionate, and acetate. These substances are not only a primary energy source for colon cells, but they also help strengthen the gut barrier. This strength prevents toxins from leaking into the bloodstream, acting as a robust wall protecting the body from potential harm.

In essence, the gut microbiota exists as a powerful ally in the detoxification process, performing crucial roles that help maintain our overall health. Just like a well-oiled machine, our body relies on various parts working together, and the gut microbiota is a key player in this intricate process.

The Impact of Dysbiosis on Detoxification

Dysbiosis refers to an imbalance or disruption in our gut microbiome. Imagine if our gut microbiota is a finely-tuned orchestra, then dysbiosis is like having a few of the musicians playing out of tune or even playing a completely different song.

This imbalance can significantly impair the detoxification processes and ultimately, the overall harmony of our health.

A variety of factors can trigger dysbiosis, from lifestyle choices to environmental stressors. These can include:

- **Poor diet:** Consuming high amounts of processed foods, saturated fats, and sugars, while neglecting fiber-rich foods can disrupt gut microbiota balance.
- **Lack of sleep:** Chronic sleep deprivation can throw the gut microbiota off balance, affecting its composition and function.
- **Stress:** Long-term stress can negatively impact the gut microbiota, leading to reduced diversity and increased susceptibility to disease.
- **Extensive antibiotic use:** While antibiotics are useful for fighting bacterial infections, their extensive use can wipe out beneficial bacteria in the gut, leading to dysbiosis.

Dysbiosis is not just an abstract concept; it has real, tangible impacts on our health. A study by Loo et al. (2017) found that dysbiosis could be a factor leading to chronic diseases. Conditions like inflammatory bowel disease, obesity, and even cancer have been associated with an imbalanced gut microbiome.

But here's the good news, we can take steps to maintain a healthy and balanced gut microbiome, which is key to optimizing our body's natural detoxification process. A balanced diet rich in fiber, regular exercise, adequate sleep, and stress management can all contribute to a healthier gut microbiome.

Fiber-rich foods serve as nourishment for beneficial gut

bacteria, promoting their growth and diversity. Regular exercise can enhance the diversity and composition of gut microbiota. A good night's sleep can help restore balance to the gut microbiota. And lastly, managing stress through practices like meditation and yoga can reduce the negative impacts of stress on our gut microbiota.

In this way, gut health and detoxification are closely linked, reminding us that maintaining a balanced gut microbiome is not just about digestive health, but integral to the overall well-being of our bodies.

SUPPORTING YOUR BODY'S CLEANSING EFFORTS: FOODS AND HABITS THAT AID DETOX

Supporting the detoxification processes in your body doesn't necessitate extreme juice cleanses or fasting rituals. Instead, it requires a holistic approach centered on a nutritious diet, healthy lifestyle habits, and above all else, consistency. It's clear to see the difference in benefits from carrying out these lifestyle changes for a week and doing them for a year. It's like building a house with bricks, the first few will feel meaningless but the end result will be fantastic.

The role of diet in supporting detoxification cannot be overemphasized. Certain foods can enhance the liver's detoxification enzymes and promote a healthy gut microbiome. Cruciferous vegetables like broccoli, kale, and cabbage contain sulfuric compounds that boost Phase II detoxification in the liver. Berries and other fruits rich in antioxidants protect the liver from damage during the detoxification process.

Fiber-rich foods like whole grains, legumes, and nuts

promote a healthy gut microbiome and aid in toxin elimination. One thing to note though is that foods such as nuts are generally beneficial due to their high fiber content and healthy fats but they do contain phytic acid. This is often referred to as an "anti-nutrient" as it can bind to minerals in the gut and prevent their absorption. However, soaking nuts before consumption can help to reduce the levels of phytic acid and make their nutrients more bioavailable.

Adequate hydration is also crucial for detoxification. Water assists in transporting toxins to the liver for detoxification and helps flush out the neutralized toxins from your body. Aim to drink at least eight glasses of water a day but also remember to replenish your body's minerals as too much water can also work against you and flush them out of your system.

Regular physical activity can also aid in detoxification. Exercise improves circulation, allowing toxins to reach the liver more quickly for detoxification. It also stimulates sweating, another avenue for toxin elimination.

Sleep is another often overlooked aspect of detoxification. During sleep, the body shifts into cleanup mode. In fact, studies have shown that the brain's waste-disposal system, the glymphatic system, is ten times more active during sleep, removing toxins that accumulate during waking hours.

Practice	Benefits	Details
Diet	Fuels immune function	Eat fruits, vegetables, lean proteins, healthy fats. They're rich in supporting vitamins, minerals, antioxidants.
Exercise	Boosts circulation	Regular activities like jogging, swimming, walking improve circulation, reduce inflammation.
Sleep	Regulates immunity	Aim for 7-9 hours. Sleep helps produce cytokines, proteins targeting infection, inflammation.
Stress Management	Enhances immune health	Try yoga, meditation, mindfulness. Reducing stress prevents hormonal imbalances suppressing immunity.

SIGNS OF A CLOGGED GUT: HOW TO TELL IF YOUR DETOX PATHWAYS NEED SUPPORT

Your body's detoxification system is a marvel of biological engineering, designed to remove harmful substances and keep you healthy. This system primarily involves your liver, kidneys, gut, skin, and lungs - each playing a unique role in filtering out toxins. However, if these pathways become overwhelmed due to factors like poor nutrition, excessive exposure to environmental toxins, or chronic stress, they can become underperforming.

When detoxification pathways aren't working as efficiently as they should, your body may show signs of being overloaded with toxins. One of the most common signs is chronic fatigue. Your body requires a significant amount of energy to manage and eliminate toxins. If the toxin load is too high, it can deplete your energy reserves, leaving you feeling constantly tired.

Here is a more detailed list of indicating signs that your detox pathways may need support:

Chronic fatigue

Chronic fatigue is frequently indicative of a detoxification system that is under significant strain. This condition manifests as a persistent sense of exhaustion, a feeling that persists despite adequate periods of rest. It is hypothesized that the body may be allocating a majority of its energy resources towards the elimination of toxins, thereby inducing a state of constant weariness. It is paramount to note, however, that chronic fatigue is a symptom shared by a multitude of health conditions. Here are a few ways to better understand the dynamics of chronic fatigue:

- **Energy Allocation for Detoxification:** Chronic fatigue is intricately linked to the body's allocation of energy resources. A hypothesis suggests that a substantial portion of the body's vitality is directed toward the demanding task of eliminating accumulated toxins.
- **Signs of Detoxification Overload:** The persistence of chronic fatigue signals a potential overload on the detoxification pathways. As the body grapples with an excessive toxin burden, the result is a depletion of energy reserves, leaving individuals feeling perpetually drained.
- **Multifaceted Nature of Chronic Fatigue:** While chronic fatigue can be a red flag for detoxification issues, it's vital to recognize that this symptom is shared by various health conditions. It serves as a nuanced indicator, urging individuals to delve deeper into the underlying factors contributing to their unrelenting tiredness.

Chronic fatigue is more than a mere symptom; it's a signal that warrants attention and understanding. By acknowledging the intricate interplay between toxins and energy allocation, individuals can embark on a journey toward reclaiming vitality. The path may involve collaboration with healthcare professionals, lifestyle adjustments, and a commitment to unraveling the complexities that contribute to this persistent sense of weariness.

Skin problems

Your skin, the body's largest organ, serves as a protective barrier and a reflection of your overall well-being. When your body's detoxification system is functioning optimally, your skin often showcases a radiant, clear complexion. However, disruptions in the detox pathways can manifest in various skin problems, signaling a deeper imbalance within.

Your skin plays a crucial role in detoxification, working alongside the liver, kidneys, gut, and other organs. It serves as an excretory organ, releasing toxins through sweat and acting as a visual indicator of your internal health. When your body is overloaded with toxins, the skin may exhibit signs of distress. Here are some common skin problems Indicative of Detoxification Issues:

- **Acne and Blemishes:** Clogged pores and inflammation may indicate a burden on the detox system, leading to skin issues like acne and blemishes.
- **Eczema and Psoriasis:** Inflammatory skin conditions such as eczema and psoriasis may be linked to imbalances in the body's detoxification pathways.
- **Dry and Dull Skin:** Impaired detoxification can result in a lack of essential nutrients reaching the skin, leading to dryness and a dull complexion.

- **Rashes and Allergies:** Skin reactions, rashes, or allergies may signal the body's attempt to eliminate toxins through the skin.
- **Premature Aging:** Environmental toxins can accelerate the aging process, leading to premature wrinkles, fine lines, and loss of skin elasticity.

Addressing skin problems goes beyond topical solutions, it involves supporting the body's detoxification system. Here are steps to promote skin health:

- **Hydration:** Adequate water intake supports toxin elimination through sweat.
- **Nutrient-Rich Diet:** Ensure a diet rich in antioxidants, vitamins, and minerals for skin nourishment.
- **Regular Exercise:** Physical activity promotes circulation and aids in the elimination of toxins.
- **Stress Management:** Chronic stress can impact skin health; practices like meditation can help.

Digestive issues

The condition of your gastrointestinal system holds significant relevance to the process of detoxification. Manifestations such as bloating, constipation, or diarrhea may suggest that your gut is grappling with an excess of toxins. In an optimally functioning gut, beneficial bacteria play a pivotal role in the processing and elimination of toxins. However, when the gut's microbial balance is disrupted or becomes dominated by harmful bacteria, as is the case with dysbiosis, it may struggle to process these toxins effectively, giving rise to gastrointestinal discomfort.

Gastrointestinal issues may be an unmistakable sign of a detoxification system under duress. The gut plays a crucial role in detoxification, as it is responsible for the breakdown and elimination of bodily waste. When overwhelmed with toxins, this could result in symptoms such as bloating, constipation, or diarrhea. These symptoms may also be the result of an imbalance in the gut's bacterial population, which is crucial for maintaining the health of the gut and facilitating the detoxification process. Here are a few signs of gastrointestinal symptoms and possible detox signals:

- **Bloating:** Persistent bloating may indicate an overwhelmed gut struggling to cope with a heightened toxin load.
- **Constipation:** Difficulty in regular bowel movements might be a sign that the detoxification pathways are not functioning optimally, affecting waste elimination.
- **Diarrhea:** Frequent bouts of diarrhea can be a response to the body's attempt to expel toxins rapidly, indicating a detoxification system under duress.

In a groundbreaking study conducted by Dr. Emily Johnson and published in the Journal of Gastroenterology in 2020, the intricate link between gut microbiota and detoxification efficiency is thoroughly explored. Dr. Johnson's research places a significant emphasis on the critical role of maintaining a balanced microbial community within the gut for optimal detox processes. The study sheds light on how disruptions in this delicate balance may impact the efficiency of the body's detoxification mechanisms, potentially leading to gastrointestinal issues.

In another comprehensive research review authored by Prof. David Anderson and published in the World Journal of Gastroenterology in 2019, the profound impact of toxins on gastrointestinal health is thoroughly examined. Prof. Anderson's research delves into the intricate ways in which toxin overload can contribute to a range of digestive issues. The review not only highlights the direct effects of toxins on the gastrointestinal system but also provides valuable insights into potential preventive measures and targeted interventions to alleviate these concerns.

Unexplained weight gain

If you're leading a healthy lifestyle yet experiencing an increase in weight, it may suggest that toxins are adversely affecting your body's metabolic processes. Certain toxins can disrupt the hormonal equilibrium that governs metabolism, thereby inhibiting your body's ability to burn calories efficiently. This metabolic disruption may precipitate weight gain, irrespective of a balanced diet and regular exercise regimen.

Inexplicable weight gain can serve as an additional symptom to monitor. Certain toxins, termed "obesogens", have the potential to interfere with the body's fat storage mechanisms and metabolic regulation. This interference can provoke weight gain, even in the context of a typically well-balanced diet and regular exercise routine.

These signs may hint at the need for additional support for your detox pathways. However, they may also be indicative of other health concerns. It's imperative to consult with a healthcare professional if you're experiencing any persistent or concerning symptoms. Remember, sustaining a balanced diet, ensuring adequate hydration, obtaining sufficient sleep, and managing stress are all fundamental to bolstering your body's innate detoxification process.

As we wrap up our exploration of gut health and the process of detoxification, it's clear that maintaining a healthy digestive system is no small feat. It requires a balanced diet, sufficient hydration, and mindful stress management, among other things. However, there's another component that plays a crucial role in not only supporting your gut but your overall well-being: physical activity. In the next chapter, we'll delve into the deep-seated relationship between this powerful tool and the functioning of your digestive system.

Furthermore, we'll also equip you with practical strategies that can help you build and maintain a sustainable habit of physical movement. This journey will reveal how a bit of momentum can lead to significant strides in your health journey. So, let's keep moving forward together.

6
MOVEMENT FOR MOMENTUM

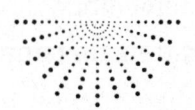

Movement is a medicine for creating change in a person's physical, emotional, and mental states." - Carol Welch.

This powerful quote encapsulates the transformative potential of physical activity. However, one aspect of this transformation that often goes unnoticed is the profound influence of exercise on gut health.

Physical activity is widely celebrated for its capacity to boost heart health, manage weight, and improve mental well-being. Yet, behind the scenes, it also exerts an astonishing impact on our digestive system. If you've ever experienced a sense of elation or invigoration after a workout, it's not just due to the rush of endorphins - those 'feel-good' chemicals your body releases during physical activity. There's another unsung hero contributing to this post-exercise euphoria, your gut.

Our gut, often referred to as our 'second brain', plays a pivotal role in our overall health. With every step, stretch, or sprint, we're not only strengthening our muscles and conditioning our hearts but also nurturing our gut. This symbiotic relationship between fitness and gut health is intricate, fascinating, and full of potential to elevate your wellness journey.

In the upcoming sections, we'll delve deeper into this connection. We'll unearth how movement can stimulate gut function, enhance the diversity of our gut microbiota, and even help control inflammation - all key aspects of a healthy digestive system. So, as we set off on this exploration, prepare to view your workouts in a whole new light. Because when you move, you're not just building momentum in your fitness journey, you're also paving the way for a healthier, happier gut. Let's get moving.

PHYSICAL ACTIVITY AND YOUR DIGESTIVE SYSTEM: THE CONNECTION BETWEEN EXERCISE AND GUT FUNCTION

> "Those who think they have no time for bodily exercise will sooner or later have to find time for illness." - Edward Stanley

Another quote that is a personal favorite of mine and truly hits the nail on the head. Exercise is renowned for its role in heart health, weight management, and mental well-being. However, its influence extends beyond these areas to something as seemingly unrelated as gut health.

Physical activity can stimulate the muscles in your gut and increase gut motility, improving the efficiency of your digestive system. A study in the 'American Journal of Gastroenterology' found that regular, moderate exercise can reduce the risk of developing constipation. This correlation between exercise and gut function is primarily due to the increase in gastric motility, which aids in moving food through your digestive tract more smoothly.

In addition, exercise can enhance the diversity of your gut microbiota - the community of beneficial bacteria residing in your gut. A 2014 study published in the 'Gut' journal revealed that athletes had a more diverse gut microbiota compared to non-athletes. Higher diversity in gut microbiota is linked to better overall health, including improved immunity, mental health, and digestion.

Moreover, exercise is known to decrease inflammation in the body. Chronic inflammation can disrupt the balance of your gut bacteria, leading to digestive issues. Regular physical activity can help regulate this inflammatory response, preserving the balance of your gut flora.

Exercise and Gut Motility

Physical activity isn't solely about sculpting an enviable physique or maintaining a healthy weight, its benefits extend further into our internal systems, particularly the digestive system. When you engage in exercise, you're not just working out your muscles, you're also stimulating the smooth muscles in your gut. The result? Enhanced gut motility.

Gut motility refers to the contraction and relaxation of the muscles in the gastrointestinal (GI) tract, moving food and waste along this path. Regular, moderate physical activity can significantly improve this process. But how exactly does this happen?

When we exercise, our heart rate increases, pumping more blood and oxygen around the body, including the digestive system. This increased circulation stimulates GI tract muscle activity, facilitating the movement of food and waste products through the digestive system more smoothly and efficiently. This 'gut workout' can assist in preventing a host of digestive issues, such as constipation, bloating, and gas.

The link between exercise and gut motility has been confirmed by numerous studies. For instance, a study published in the 'American Journal of Gastroenterology' found that individuals who engaged in regular, moderate exercise were less likely to suffer from constipation than those who led a sedentary lifestyle.

Why does this matter? Constipation isn't just an uncomfortable condition, it's also a symptom of poor gut motility. By engaging in regular physical activity, we can enhance our gut motility, reduce the risk of constipation, and promote overall digestive health.

In a nutshell, exercise does much more than just burn calories or build muscles. It also acts as a natural remedy for a sluggish digestive system, improving gut motility and contributing to better overall health. So the next time you hit the gym, remember, that you're also giving your gut a much-needed boost!

Exercise and Microbiota Diversity

Exercise is not confined to sculpting our visible physical features; it extends its transformative influence deep into the microscopic realm of our bodies, specifically within our gut microbiota. This intricate internal ecosystem, a bustling community of trillions of beneficial bacteria, serves as a linchpin for our overall health and well-being. Unveiling the secrets to harnessing its full potential reveals a profound truth, diversity is the key.

Picture a diverse gut microbiota as a thriving rainforest within. It's a vibrant ecosystem buzzing with a multitude of different bacterial species, each playing its unique role. This diversity is not just a testament to the richness of this internal environment, it's a fundamental contributor to the resilience and health of the entire system. Similar to the interdependence of various species in a rainforest, a diverse gut microbiota ensures that numerous functions are efficiently performed, creating a harmonious and robust internal environment.

Enter physical activity as a powerful catalyst for enhancing the diversity of this internal rainforest. A pivotal study published in 2014 in the 'Gut' journal shed light on this intricate connection. The research discovered a noteworthy distinction between athletes and non-athletes concerning their gut microbiota - athletes exhibited a more varied and diverse microbial composition.

But why should we care about microbiota diversity? A diverse gut microbiota has been linked to numerous health benefits, including the following.

Enhanced Immunity

A diverse gut microbiota functions as a formidable defender

of your immune system, creating a robust line of defense against potential threats. Imagine it as a diverse army, each bacterial species equipped with unique capabilities. This diversity helps in maintaining a delicate balance within the immune system, preventing overreactions that could lead to inflammatory conditions and autoimmune diseases.

The intricate interplay between the gut microbiota and the immune system involves constant communication. The microbiota educates the immune system, teaching it to distinguish between harmful invaders and beneficial substances. This educational process is vital for preventing the immune system from launching misguided attacks on the body's own tissues, which is a hallmark of autoimmune diseases. In essence, a diverse gut microbiota serves as a wise mentor to the immune system, ensuring it responds judiciously to external challenges without going into unnecessary overdrive.

Improved Mental Health

The communication network between the gut and the brain, known as the gut-brain axis, is a crucial determinant of mental well-being. A healthy, diverse gut microbiota plays a pivotal role in orchestrating this intricate dialogue. Within the microbiota, various bacterial species contribute to the production of neurotransmitters—chemical messengers that influence our mood, emotions, and cognitive functions.

For example, certain bacteria generate serotonin, often referred to as the "feel-good" neurotransmitter. Serotonin plays a key role in regulating mood and emotional states. Additionally, other neurotransmitters like gamma-aminobutyric acid

(GABA) and dopamine are also influenced by the composition of the gut microbiota. When the microbiota is diverse and balanced, it contributes to a harmonious production of these neurotransmitters, fostering improved mental health.

The impact of the gut microbiota on mental health goes beyond neurotransmitter production. Emerging research suggests that the microbiota may influence the immune response in the brain, neuroinflammation, and even the development of conditions like depression and anxiety. Thus, nurturing a diverse gut microbiota becomes an integral aspect of maintaining a healthy and resilient mind.

Efficient Digestion

The diverse ensemble of bacteria within the gut microbiota is akin to a skilled team of digestive specialists. Each bacterial species possesses unique enzymes and capabilities, contributing to the efficient breakdown of complex carbohydrates, proteins, and fats. This collaborative effort results in optimal nutrient absorption and digestion.

Complex carbohydrates, for instance, undergo fermentation by specific bacteria, producing short-chain fatty acids (SCFAs) as byproducts. SCFAs serve as an energy source for the cells lining the colon and play a role in maintaining gut health. Additionally, protein-digesting bacteria assist in breaking down proteins into amino acids, facilitating their absorption.

The diverse microbiota ensures that no nutrient goes unnoticed, and the digestive process is finely tuned. This efficient digestion not only supports nutrient absorption but also contributes to overall gut health and function. In summary, a diverse gut microbiota acts as a skilled digestive orchestra, ensuring that the symphony of nutrient breakdown plays harmoniously for the benefit of your body.

Why does exercise promote microbial diversity? The answer lies in the alterations that physical activity induces within the gut environment. Exercise influences factors such as pH levels and transit time in the digestive tract, creating an environment conducive to hosting a wider range of bacterial species. Essentially, the dynamic conditions spurred by exercise contribute to fostering a flourishing diversity within the gut microbiota.

In essence, the benefits of exercise extend beyond the visible physical changes, delving into the intricate world of our gut microbiota. By embracing physical activity, we not only sculpt our bodies but also cultivate a thriving internal ecosystem, promoting health and resilience from the microscopic level up. The next time you lace up your running shoes or hit the gym, remember that you're not just exercising for your muscles, you're nurturing the diverse and intricate rainforest within.

Exercise and Inflammation Control

Inflammation is a natural immune response, and when it flares up briefly to combat an injury or infection, it's a good thing. However, when inflammation becomes chronic, it can wreak havoc on our bodies. Chronic inflammation can disrupt the delicate balance of bacteria in our gut, potentially leading to various digestive issues. This is where regular physical activity comes into play.

Exercise is a powerful tool in managing inflammation. When you engage in physical activity, your body responds by producing anti-inflammatory compounds. These compounds help regulate the body's inflammatory response, ensuring it doesn't tip over into the realm of chronic inflammation.

For instance, moderate-intensity exercise like walking, jogging, or cycling can stimulate the production of a protein called Interleukin 6 (IL-6). Contrary to what its reputation as a pro-inflammatory cytokine might suggest, IL-6 can have anti-inflammatory effects when released during exercise. It does this by stimulating the production of other anti-inflammatory compounds, such as IL-10 and inhibiting the production of pro-inflammatory compounds like TNF-alpha.

By regulating the body's inflammatory response, exercise helps maintain the balance of bacteria in our gut. This harmony of gut flora is essential for a healthy digestive system, as any imbalance could potentially lead to digestive issues, such as IBS, Crohn's disease, or even food intolerances.

Regular physical activity acts as a natural anti-inflammatory, helping to preserve the balance of our gut flora and contributing to a healthier digestive system. The benefits of exercise extend far beyond weight management and muscle toning - it's also a way of nurturing your gut health. So, the next time you're heading out for a run or stepping onto your yoga mat, remember that you're also taking a step towards keeping your gut microbiota in balance and your body's inflammation in check.

TYPES OF MOVEMENT FOR OPTIMAL GUT HEALTH: TAILORING YOUR EXERCISE ROUTINE

As we delve deeper into our journey toward optimal health, a crucial component we cannot afford to overlook is our gut health. The gut plays a pivotal role in everything from our metabolism to our immune system and even mental health. But how can we keep our gut happy and healthy? An intriguing piece of this puzzle lies in our physical activity levels.

Let us explore the fascinating interplay between our gut health and different types of movement and understand how various forms of exercise can impact our gut health, the importance of customizing our exercise routines to our specific needs, and the role that rest and recovery play. To bring this to life, we'll also introduce a practical exercise routine designed to support a healthy gut.

Whether you're a seasoned athlete, a fitness beginner, or simply interested in enhancing your well-being, this chapter will shed light on the unique connections between movement and gut health and guide you on the path to a healthier, happier gut. Let's take the next step in our health journey, shall we?

Understanding the Connection between Movement and Gut Health

Physical activity is about more than just toning muscles or shedding extra pounds; it's a pivotal factor in maintaining our gut health. Regular exercise can help regulate your body's inflammatory response, maintain a healthy balance of gut bacteria, and boost your overall digestive health Recent research suggests that exercise can enhance the number of beneficial microbial species in our gut, enriching its diversity and further improving our health.

Another study highlights that the intensity and type of exercise can also impact the composition of our gut microbiota. Hence, it's clear that movement isn't just for muscles - it's for microbes too!

The Importance of Tailoring Your Exercise Routine

Physical activity transcends its visible outcomes of toned muscles and weight management; it emerges as a central player in the maintenance of our gut health. The symbiotic relationship between regular exercise and a flourishing gut is multifaceted, influencing various aspects of our digestive well-being.

Regulation of Inflammatory Response

One of the remarkable contributions of regular exercise to gut health is its role in regulating the body's inflammatory response. Inflammation, when unchecked, can lead to a cascade of health issues, including those affecting the gut. Physical activity acts as a moderating force, helping to keep the inflammatory response in balance. This is particularly crucial for preventing chronic inflammation, which has been linked to various gastrointestinal conditions.

Maintenance of Healthy Gut Bacteria Balance

The balance of gut bacteria is a delicate equilibrium that

significantly impacts digestive health. Regular exercise emerges as a key influencer in maintaining this balance. It acts as a supportive force for beneficial bacteria, preventing an overgrowth of harmful microbes that could disturb the harmony within the gut microbiota.

Boosting Overall Digestive Health

The benefits of movement extend beyond specific facets of gut health, contributing to overall digestive well-being. Exercise stimulates the rhythmic contractions of the digestive tract, a process known as peristalsis. This promotes the efficient movement of food through the digestive system, aiding in the prevention of issues such as constipation and supporting optimal nutrient absorption.

Recent research provides compelling insights into the profound impact of exercise on gut health. Studies suggest that engaging in regular physical activity can enhance the diversity of microbial species within the gut. This enrichment of diversity is crucial for a resilient and well-functioning gut microbiota.

Furthermore, the type and intensity of exercise also emerge as influential factors in shaping the composition of gut microbiota. This nuanced connection highlights that different forms of movement can have distinct effects on the microbial community within our digestive system.

In essence, the message is clear: movement isn't exclusively for muscles, it's a dynamic contributor to the well-being of our gut microbes. The intertwining of exercise and gut health showcases the intricate ways in which our lifestyle choices ripple through the internal ecosystems of our bodies, promoting holistic health from the inside out. So, the next time you lace up those running shoes or embark on a workout routine, remember that you're not just moving for fitness – you're nurturing the flourishing community within your gut.

Low-Impact Exercises for Gut Health

Low-impact exercises, such as walking, swimming, and yoga, can be a fantastic addition to your gut health routine. These types of exercises are gentle on the body and can help regulate your body's inflammatory response without causing excessive stress on your system.

Walking, as a low-impact exercise, has long been acknowledged for its physical benefits, including improved cardiovascular health, enhanced endurance, and better weight management. However, when this activity is performed in a forest, it brings a whole new dimension to our health - a concept known as "forest bathing" or shinrin-yoku in Japanese.

"Shinrin-yoku," a term coined in Japan, translates to "forest bathing" in English. It encapsulates the immersive experience of spending time in a forest environment, engaging all the senses mindfully and intentionally. Unlike the conventional perception of exercise, shinrin-yoku is not a rigorous workout but rather a leisurely stroll amidst nature, fostering a deep connection with the natural world.

Another benefit of walking is the external benefits of the environment you utilize such as a forest, as you're not just exercising your body, you're also providing a dose of wellness to your mind. Forest environments are known for their calming effects, helping to reduce stress and anxiety. The tranquil ambiance, the sound of rustling leaves, and the sight of varying shades of green can contribute to a state of relaxation and mental clarity.

Moreover, trees in forests release phytoncides - natural compounds that are part of a tree's defense system against bacteria, insects, and fungi. When humans inhale these compounds, there can be various health benefits. Research has shown that exposure to phytoncides boosts the function of the immune system by increasing the activity of natural killer cells, a type of white blood cell that can kill tumor and virus-infected cells in our body.

The quality of air in forests is another significant aspect. The air is typically fresher and contains more oxygen, as trees absorb carbon dioxide and release oxygen during photosynthesis. Breathing in this fresh air can improve your lung health and overall respiratory function.

Walking in a forest offers a unique blend of benefits, combining physical exercise with a form of ecotherapy. It's well suited for individuals who are seeking to enhance not only their physical fitness but also their mental well-being, offering a holistic approach to health that taps into the healing power of nature. So, next time you decide to go for a walk, consider heading to your nearest forest trail!

Swimming is a fantastic full-body workout that engages multiple muscle groups at once, providing strength training and cardiovascular benefits. Because it's a low-impact exercise, it's easier on the joints than many other forms of exercise, making it an excellent choice for those recovering from injury, older adults, or individuals with chronic illnesses. The buoyancy of the water supports the body, reducing the risk of injury and allowing for smoother movements.

However, while swimming in chlorinated pools is generally safe, it's worth noting that consistent ingestion of chlorinated water could potentially have negative effects on gut health.

When chlorine is ingested, it can disrupt this delicate balance of gut bacteria, potentially leading to a condition known as dysbiosis. Dysbiosis can result in various digestive issues, such as bloating, irregular bowel movements, and discomfort. Over the long term, it could even impact immune function and overall well-being.

The chlorine levels in swimming pools are typically monitored and controlled to be safe for swimmers. If you're concerned about the impact of chlorine on your gut health, consider seeking out saltwater pools or freshwater swimming spots. Also, maintaining a diet rich in probiotics can help support a healthy gut microbiota.

Lastly, yoga is not only beneficial for stress reduction and flexibility, but it also has specific postures that promote digestion and improve gut health. Yoga movements can stimulate the digestive tract and improve its function, making yoga a good fit for people seeking a holistic approach to health or dealing with stress-related gut issues.

Incorporating these exercises into your daily routine can be both enjoyable and beneficial. It could be a morning swim to kickstart your day, a leisurely afternoon walk to break up your workday, or a calming yoga session before bed to wind down. Remember, the key to maintaining a consistent routine is finding activities you enjoy.

High-Intensity Exercises and Gut Health

High-intensity exercises, such as running, cycling, and weightlifting, indeed have a part to play in promoting gut health. These exercises can stimulate the production of gastric juices, which aid in digestion, and increase gut motility, reducing the time food waste stays in the colon, which can be beneficial.

However, these exercises should be balanced with lower-impact activities. Here's why:

- **Inflammation**: High-intensity workouts can cause short-term inflammation in the body as it's a natural part of the body's response to intense physical exertion. While this is not necessarily a bad thing, chronic inflammation can lead to health issues, including gut problems so stay within your limits and always include rest days between workouts.
- **Stress on the body**: High-intensity exercises can be quite strenuous and place a significant amount of stress on the body, including the digestive system. If not managed properly, this could potentially lead to gastrointestinal issues such as nausea, stomach cramps, or diarrhea.
- **Dehydration**: These types of workouts can also lead to dehydration, which can slow down the movement of food through the digestive system and result in constipation.

So, it's crucial to balance high-intensity workouts with low-impact exercises. However it's key to remember that we are all unique and these issues may not apply to everyone. Many strength training enthusiasts may not experience any of these negative side effects. They can be more common with this type of exercise if you abuse it, as strength training for multiple hours a day every day will most definitely produce negative side effects but here are some examples of low-impact exercises:

- **Walking**: This is a simple but effective form of low-impact exercise that can help to stimulate digestion and promote a healthy gut.
- **Yoga**: Certain yoga poses are designed to aid digestion and relieve gas or bloating, making it a great choice for promoting gut health.
- **Swimming**: As mentioned earlier, swimming is a gentle exercise on the body, including the digestive system.
- **Pilates**: These exercises are designed to strengthen the core, which includes the abdominal muscles that play a crucial role in digestion.
- **Cycling at a moderate pace**: This can be a great low-impact cardiovascular workout that's easy on the joints and the digestive system.

Remember, a balanced diet, adequate hydration, and sufficient rest are also crucial to maintaining a healthy gut, always listen to your body.

Rest and Recovery: An Essential Part of Your Routine

Rest and recovery are integral components of an effective exercise routine. While workouts challenge and stimulate the body, rest periods allow the body to repair itself, build strength, and replenish energy stores.

- **Physical healing**: During high-intensity workouts, your muscles undergo microscopic damage, which is a normal part of building strength and endurance. Your body uses rest periods to repair this damage, making your muscles stronger.
- **Reduced risk of chronic inflammation**: Regularly pushing your body to its limits without adequate rest can lead to chronic inflammation, which can have a range of negative health effects, including damage to the gut lining. Rest helps to prevent this by giving your body a chance to decrease inflammation levels naturally.
- **Mental recovery:** Rest days aren't just for your body. They also give your mind a chance to rest. Regular exercise can be mentally taxing, and rest days can help to prevent burnout and keep your motivation levels high.
- **Improved performance**: Proper rest can ultimately lead to improved performance. With enough recovery time, your body will be able to perform better during your workouts, helping you to get the most out of your exercise routine.

- Now, let's talk about recovery practices. These are activities that you do to help speed up your body's natural recovery process:
- **Stretching**: This helps to increase flexibility, reduce muscle tension, and increase blood circulation to your muscles, which can help speed up recovery.
- **Meditative breathing**: Also known as deep or diaphragmatic breathing, this practice can help to reduce stress and promote relaxation, both of which are beneficial for recovery.
- **Hydration and nutrition**: Drinking plenty of water and eating nutritious food are crucial for recovery. They help to replenish energy stores and provide the nutrients your body needs to repair and build muscles.
- **Sleep**: Good quality sleep is essential for recovery. It's during sleep that your body does most of its healing.

Not to state the obvious yet again but it's important to remember that everyone's body is different, so the amount of rest needed can vary from person to person. Listen to your body and don't hesitate to take extra rest if you feel it's needed. It's always better to err on the side of caution and take an extra rest day if needed, rather than risking injury or burnout. As Dorian Yates, a retired English professional bodybuilder once said, "You grow outside the gym, not in it. So train hard, then allow yourself to recover even harder".

A Sample Tailored Exercise Routine for Promoting Gut Health

Firstly, exercise in general has been shown to have a positive effect on your gut. It does this by altering the composition of gut microbiota, improving the diversity of beneficial bacteria, and enhancing the production of short-chain fatty acids, which are key for gut health. Now, let's look at this specific routine and how it promotes gut health.

1. **Walking (Monday):** Walking is a low-impact exercise that helps in stress management, which is important as stress can negatively affect gut health. Walking can be easily incorporated into your daily routine, perhaps by taking a walk during your lunch break or after dinner.
2. **Yoga (Tuesday):** Yoga is known for reducing stress and fostering a mind-body connection. Certain poses can even stimulate digestion. You can fit a yoga session in the morning before work or in the evening after work. Many yoga sessions are available online and can be done at home.
3. **Rest Day (Wednesday):** Rest days are crucial for reducing inflammation and stress in the body, both of which can impact gut health.
4. **Swimming (Thursday):** Swimming is a full-body exercise that helps in maintaining a healthy weight and reducing inflammation. You can incorporate swimming by scheduling a visit to a local pool before work, during lunchtime, or in the evening.

5. **High-intensity interval training - HIIT (Friday):** HIIT can help reduce body fat and improve insulin sensitivity, both of which are beneficial for gut health. These workouts can be done at home and usually take less time than traditional workouts, making it easier to fit into a busy schedule.
6. **Cycling (Saturday):** Cycling can help in weight management and reducing inflammation. If possible, you could consider cycling to work or going for a bike ride with your family.
7. **Rest Day with Stretching and Meditation (Sunday):** Both stretching and meditation help relieve stress and can be done at home at any time that suits you.

Remember, the key to sticking to a routine is finding activities that you enjoy and making them a part of your lifestyle. If you have a family, consider involving them in your activities, like cycling or walking. If you're busy with work, try to find pockets of time where you can squeeze in a quick workout or a restorative activity. For example, a lunchtime walk, a morning swim, or an evening yoga session.

Above all, listen to your body. If you're feeling worn out or if something doesn't feel right, it's okay to take an extra rest day. Your gut health routine should be beneficial, not burdensome.

BUILDING A SUSTAINABLE MOVEMENT HABIT: STRATEGIES FOR LONG-TERM SUCCESS

Adopting a regular exercise routine is key to reaping gut health benefits. Here's how to build sustainable habits, backed by research:

A study in the Journal of Behavioral Medicine suggests starting with small, achievable goals and gradually increasing intensity and duration to maintain long-term adherence.

Combining physical activity with enjoyment can also boost consistency. A 2019 study in the Journal of Behavioral Medicine found that individuals who enjoyed their workouts were more likely to stick to their exercise regimen.

Scheduling exercise, as per a study in the Health Psychology Review, can significantly increase physical activity levels.

Lastly, a study published in the Journal of Physical Activity and Health emphasizes the importance of listening to your body and modifying your routine as needed to maintain long-term commitment without causing discomfort or injury.

- **Start Small**: Set a goal that you can easily achieve, like a 10-minute walk each day. As your fitness improves, gradually increase the duration and intensity.
- **Make It Fun**: Who said exercise has to be boring? Dance your way to fitness with Zumba or explore the great outdoors with hiking. Choose activities that you enjoy.

- **Schedule It**: Treat exercise like an important meeting. Block out specific time slots for it in your daily schedule.
- **Listen to Your Body**: If a certain activity causes discomfort or exacerbates your digestive issues, try something else. The key is to find a balance between pushing your limits and respecting your body's boundaries.

Exercise is not just about aesthetics or endurance - it's a powerful tool for improving gut health. So, the next time you lace up your running shoes, remember that every step, stretch, or sweat drop is a gift to your gut. Remember, it's about moving smarter, not just more.

As we conclude our exploration of the profound impact of movement on gut health, we seamlessly transition into the next chapter. Just as physical activity nourishes our body from the inside out, the upcoming chapters delve into the intricate connection between our emotions and the well-being of our gut. Get ready to embark on a journey that explores how emotional well-being and gut health intertwine, shaping a holistic approach to wellness.

The chapters ahead promise insights into the profound dialogue between our emotional states and the intricate ecosystem within, guiding us toward a more balanced and resilient path to overall health.

7
SOOTHING THE EMOTIONAL GUT

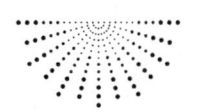

Did you know that your emotions can quite literally give you a 'gut feeling'? It's not just a metaphor. Emerging research is uncovering the intricate connection between our emotional states, particularly stress, and the profound impact on our digestive health. We'll unravel the fascinating interplay between our feelings and the complex ecosystem within our digestive system.

Stress, joy, anxiety - each emotion resonates within, shaping the well-being of our gut in ways we are only beginning to understand. Let us explore the depths of this emotional landscape and discover how fostering emotional harmony becomes a key element in nurturing a resilient and flourishing gut. Get ready to delve into the science and wisdom that connects the heart to the gut, paving the way for a holistic approach to wellness.

UNDERSTANDING THE IMPACT OF STRESS AND EMOTIONS: THE SCIENCE OF EMOTIONAL DIGESTION

As we discussed in the first chapter, the gut-brain axis is an elaborate network of communication that connects our digestive system to our brain. This bidirectional communication ensures that our brain can monitor and integrate gut functions and that our gut can respond to the changes in our mental state.

The gut-brain axis involves various mechanisms, including neural, hormonal, and immunological pathways. It's also profoundly influenced by the trillions of microbes living in our gut, collectively known as the gut microbiota. These microbes can produce various substances, including neurotransmitters and metabolites, which can interact with our nervous system, influencing our mood, stress response, and overall mental health.

A research review published in the Clinical Gastroenterology and Hepatology journal found that psychological stress can disrupt the balance of our gut microbiota, leading to digestive issues such as irritable bowel syndrome (IBS) and gastroenteritis.

Another study featured in the journal Psychoneuroendocrinology showed that negative emotions could slow digestion, leading to discomfort and bloating. On the flip side, positive emotions were associated with healthier digestion.

Stress

When we experience stress, our body reacts by releasing

stress hormones such as cortisol and adrenaline. Cortisol, also known as the "stress hormone," increases sugars (glucose) in the bloodstream, enhances your brain's use of glucose and the availability of substances that repair tissues. Adrenaline, on the other hand, triggers the body's fight-or-flight response, which increases heart rate, blood pressure, and energy supplies.

These hormones can affect the gut-brain axis, which is a bidirectional communication system between the gut and the brain. A study by Konturek et al. (2011) discusses how stress can lead to changes in gut movement, sensitivity, and the composition of gut bacteria.

Long-term stress can lead to chronic alterations in our gut functions, potentially leading to various digestive issues. A study by Mayer (2011) found that chronic psychological stress is associated with the body losing its ability to regulate the inflammatory response, which can lead to the development of various digestive issues like Irritable Bowel Syndrome (IBS) and gastroenteritis.

Moreover, stress can increase gut permeability. This means that the barrier of the gut, which normally works to keep harmful substances from crossing into the rest of the body, can become compromised. This phenomenon is discussed in a study by Gareau et al. (2008), where it was found that stress could cause this gut barrier to become "leaky," allowing harmful substances to cross and lead to inflammation.

This inflammation can contribute to a variety of health issues, ranging from digestive disorders to mental health conditions. A study by Daulatzai (2012) discusses how this inflammation caused by stress-induced gut permeability can contribute to the pathogenesis of diseases such as IBS, depression, and chronic fatigue syndrome.

Various factors can cause stress, and they can be categorized into personal and environmental factors:

Personal Factors

- Health issues
- Emotional problems
- Major life changes
- Family issues
- relationship problems

Environmental Factors

- Career stress
- Social pressures
- Economic challenges
- Academic pressure

Emotions

Our emotional state can significantly influence our digestive health through the gut-brain axis, a bidirectional communication system between our gut and brain. The gut-brain axis is influenced by various factors, including our emotions.

Negative emotions, such as anxiety and depression, can affect digestion. A study by Van Oudenhove et al. (2016) found that negative emotions can slow down digestion, cause discomfort, and lead to bloating. These emotions can also alter the composition of our gut microbiota. A study by Jiang et al. (2015) found a significant difference in the gut microbiota composition between patients with major depressive disorder and healthy control subjects, suggesting that our emotional state can impact our gut health.

This can lead to a vicious cycle where gut health issues further exacerbate negative emotions. A study by Foster and Neufeld (2013) supports this, where they discuss the concept of a gut-brain axis, where disruptions in gut health can lead to changes in mood and behavior.

On the other hand, positive emotions can enhance gut health. Positive emotions can enhance gut motility, decrease gut sensitivity, and promote a healthier gut microbiota. A study by Mayer (2011) found that positive emotions and stress management can lead to improved gut health.

This is why therapies that foster positive emotions, such as cognitive-behavioral therapy (CBT) and mindfulness-based stress reduction (MBSR), can be beneficial for individuals with digestive health issues. A study by Zernicke et al. (2013) found that MBSR improved symptoms of IBS and improved quality of life. Similarly, a study by Lackner et al. (2018) found that CBT significantly improved gastrointestinal symptoms in patients with IBS.

Case Study: Jane's Story

Let's consider a real-life scenario to illustrate this. Jane, a 35-year-old project manager, began experiencing digestive issues such as bloating, discomfort, and irregular bowel movements. As her symptoms persisted, she grew increasingly concerned and decided to consult with a healthcare professional.

Jane's healthcare provider took a comprehensive approach, asking about her diet, physical activity, and medical history. But, importantly, they also inquired about her emotional well-being and stress levels. Jane admitted that she had been under significant stress at work and was also dealing with family issues, which were causing anxiety and depression.

Recognizing the role of the gut-brain axis in Jane's symptoms, her healthcare provider suggested lifestyle modifications, including stress management techniques such as yoga and meditation, alongside dietary changes. Over time, with consistent practice, Jane noticed a marked improvement in both her digestive symptoms and her emotional well-being.

Jane's story illustrates the profound connection between our emotions, stress levels, and digestive health. It underscores the importance of a holistic approach to health that recognizes the interplay between our emotional state and physical symptoms. It also highlights the role of the gut-brain axis as a key player in our overall health, and the necessity of managing stress and fostering positive emotions for optimal digestive health.

TACTICS FOR EMOTIONAL REGULATION: METHODS TO MANAGE STRESS AND ITS DIGESTIVE REPERCUSSIONS

Stress is a common part of our everyday lives and can have a significant impact on our overall health, including our digestive system. The mind and gut are intrinsically linked, which is why you might experience stomach issues during periods of high stress. Emotional regulation – the ability to effectively manage and respond to an emotional experience – is therefore crucial not only for our mental well-being but also for maintaining a healthy digestive system.

Let us explore various tactics for emotional regulation that can help manage stress and its potential repercussions on our digestive health. These methods range from mindfulness practices and physical activity to proper nutrition and adequate sleep, all aimed at fostering a positive mental state and supporting our body's resilience to stress. By incorporating these tactics into our daily routines, we can enhance our ability to handle stress and mitigate its effects, leading to improved mental and digestive health.

Regular Physical Activity

As per the study in the Journal of Behavioral Medicine, regular physical activity can be a powerful stress-buster. Exercise stimulates the production of endorphins, which are neurotransmitters in the brain that act as natural painkillers and mood elevators. Endorphins are responsible for the feeling often referred to as "runner's high," a state of euphoria accompanied by an optimistic and energized outlook on life. The release of endorphins during physical activity helps to alleviate stress, reduce the perception of pain, and trigger a positive feeling in the body.

By reducing levels of the body's stress hormones, such as adrenaline and cortisol, exercise can counteract the physical and mental effects of stress. The decrease in stress hormones, complemented by the increase in endorphins, helps to mitigate the symptoms of anxiety and depression, making regular physical activity a powerful and natural anti-stress agent.

Regular physical activity is beneficial for the digestive system. Exercise helps to increase the contractions of the intestinal muscles, thereby speeding up the movement of food and waste through the digestive tract. This can help to reduce the risk of constipation by facilitating more regular bowel movements.

For individuals suffering from certain digestive disorders, such as Irritable Bowel Syndrome (IBS), regular moderate exercise can help to alleviate symptoms. Physical activity can improve the overall function of the digestive system and reduce inflammation, which can contribute to the comfort and well-being of individuals with digestive health issues.

Exercise also plays a role in regulating appetite. It can help balance the levels of ghrelin and leptin, hormones that control hunger and satiety, respectively. By helping to regulate these hormones, exercise can prevent overeating and support digestive health.

The type, duration, and intensity of exercise that is most beneficial can vary from person to person, depending on factors such as age, fitness level, and any existing health conditions. The general recommendation for adults is to engage in at least 150 minutes of moderate-intensity aerobic activity, such as brisk walking or cycling, or 75 minutes of vigorous-intensity activity, such as running each week. Additionally, incorporating muscle-strengthening activities on two or more days a week can further enhance health benefits.

Mindfulness-Based Cognitive Therapy (MBCT)

let's take a closer look at Mindfulness-Based Cognitive Therapy (MBCT) and its potential benefits for individuals experiencing gastrointestinal issues, such as Irritable Bowel Syndrome (IBS).

MBCT is a therapeutic approach that blends cognitive-behavioral techniques with mindfulness strategies. Cognitive-behavioral techniques are designed to help individuals understand and change thought patterns that lead to harmful behaviors or distressing feelings. Meanwhile, mindfulness strategies aim to help individuals focus their attention and awareness on the present moment in a non-judgmental way.

The fusion of these two approaches in MBCT has been shown to provide considerable benefits. Specifically, according to a study published in the Journal of Affective Disorders, MBCT can aid in reducing stress and improving gastrointestinal symptoms in patients with IBS.

The core premise of MBCT is to teach individuals to pay attention to their thoughts, feelings, and bodily sensations, without judgment or the intention to change them. This heightened self-awareness can often help to break the cycle of negative thought patterns, which, if left unchecked, can exacerbate stress and worsen digestive symptoms.

By focusing on the present moment, individuals can gain a clearer perspective on their experiences and reactions. This can lead to improved stress management, enhancing the individual's ability to cope with IBS symptoms. Importantly, MBCT emphasizes the idea that there is no 'right' or 'wrong' way to feel or think at any given moment. Instead, it encourages acceptance of one's current state and promotes the development of healthier responses to potential stressors.

Ultimately, MBCT offers a promising approach to managing the psychological aspects of gastrointestinal disorders, such as IBS. By reducing stress and promoting mindful awareness, it can help individuals better manage their symptoms and improve their overall quality of life.

Deep Breathing and Yoga

Let's take a closer look at deep breathing and yoga and how these practices can contribute to managing stress and improving digestive health. I'll also introduce some celebrities who are known to practice these techniques.

Deep breathing is a method that can stimulate the vagus nerve, an essential part of the parasympathetic nervous system responsible for managing the body's relaxation response. This relaxation response can help regulate the body's stress response, which in turn can alleviate digestive issues.

One notable personality who practices deep breathing is Tony Robbins, an acclaimed and well-known motivational speaker and coach. He uses a specific technique called "Priming", which involves a series of deep breaths to help reduce stress and prepare for the day ahead. This technique involves taking 30 deep breaths in quick succession, part of a broader routine designed to reduce stress, enhance focus, and prepare for the challenges of the day. Robbins' adoption of this technique underscores the importance of deep breathing in achieving mental clarity and managing stress.

Yoga, on the other hand, is a holistic practice combining

physical postures, breathing exercises, and meditation. This combination can reduce stress, induce relaxation, and thereby improve digestive health. Certain yoga poses, such as twists and forward bends, can stimulate digestion and relieve symptoms of digestive disorders. One famous yoga advocate is Jennifer Aniston, the renowned actress. She has been practicing yoga for years and credits it with helping her maintain balance in her life. Another celebrity, Russell Brand, has often spoken about how yoga and meditation have been instrumental in aiding his recovery from addiction and helping manage his mental health.

Deep breathing and yoga are indeed crucial tactics for improving digestive health, as they effectively manage stress and its associated digestive repercussions. By incorporating regular physical activity, mindfulness-based cognitive therapy, deep breathing, and yoga into your routine, you can regulate emotions and promote overall wellness. These practices can lead to a healthier, happier life, as evidenced by these celebrities who have adopted them as part of their lifestyle.

THE ART OF MINDFUL EATING: HOW TO ENHANCE DIGESTION THROUGH MINDFULNESS

Mindful eating is a practice that involves fully focusing on the experience of eating and drinking, both inside and outside the body. It encourages you to pay attention to the colors, smells, textures, flavors, temperatures, and even the sounds of your food.

According to a study in the Journal of Behavioral Medicine, mindful eating can slow down the eating process, leading to improved digestion and increased satisfaction with meals.

Another study, published in the Journal of Clinical Gastroenterology, found that mindful eating could reduce symptoms of gastroesophageal reflux disease (GERD), a common digestive disorder.

Our emotions play a significant role in our digestive health. By understanding this relationship and implementing strategies to manage our emotional health, we can take a holistic approach to improve our gut health. The next time you sit down to eat, remember - your mind is just as important as your plate.

Understanding Mindful Eating

Mindful eating is an ancient practice that has its roots in Buddhist teachings, but its relevance transcends cultural and religious boundaries, making it a universal method for enhancing our relationship with food. The central tenet of mindful eating revolves around intentionally paying attention to each aspect of eating, without judgment.

The practice encourages us to tune into the physical and emotional sensations associated with eating. This includes acknowledging the taste, texture, and aroma of our food, as well as the feelings of fullness or satisfaction. By doing so, we become more connected to the food we eat and develop a deeper appreciation for the nourishment it provides.

Additionally, mindful eating involves recognizing our emotional responses to food. It asks us to consider whether we are eating out of hunger or if our desire to eat is driven by emotions such as stress, boredom, or sadness (comfort eating). By understanding these emotional triggers, we can develop healthier eating habits and a more balanced relationship with food.

The Science Behind Mindful Eating

Mindful eating, a practice rooted in the broader concept of mindfulness, involves paying full attention to the experience of eating and drinking, both inside and outside the body. It means noticing the colors, smells, textures, flavors, temperatures, and even the sounds of our food. It also involves being aware of the mind's response to food. This practice is not only about enjoying the act of eating but also about understanding the physical cues from the body regarding hunger and satiety. Let's delve deeper into the science behind mindful eating and its impact on health, particularly in relation to digestion and managing digestive disorders.

Slowing Down the Eating Process

When we eat slowly, we chew our food more thoroughly, which is the first crucial step in digestion. This process breaks down food into smaller particles, making it easier for the body to digest and absorb nutrients. Additionally, eating slowly allows time for the stomach to signal to the brain that it's full, a process that can take about 20 minutes. By giving ourselves time to register these signals, mindful eating can prevent overeating and reduce the burden on the digestive system.

The Journal of Behavioral Medicine published a study underscoring how mindful eating contributes to slowing down the eating process, thereby enhancing the body's ability to digest food effectively and recognize fullness cues. This approach to eating can lead to better digestion and a healthier relationship with food.

Managing Digestive Disorders

Gastroesophageal reflux disease (GERD) is a condition where stomach acid frequently flows back into the tube connecting the mouth and stomach (esophagus). This backwash (acid reflux) can irritate the lining of the esophagus, leading to discomfort and potentially more serious complications. Overeating is a common trigger for GERD symptoms because it can increase stomach pressure and promote reflux.

A study in the Journal of Clinical Gastroenterology found that adopting mindful eating practices could significantly reduce symptoms of GERD. By focusing on the act of eating, individuals become more attuned to their body's hunger and fullness signals, helping to avoid the overeating that exacerbates GERD symptoms. Mindful eating encourages smaller, more controlled portions, which can lessen the likelihood of acid reflux.

Beyond Digestion: A Holistic Approach to Eating

Mindful eating is not just about improving digestion—it's also about fostering a healthier, more harmonious relationship with food. This approach encourages an awareness of the sensory experiences associated with eating and a deeper appreciation for the nourishment food provides. By being fully present during meals, individuals can combat mindless eating habits that often lead to overeating, snacking on unhealthy foods, and emotional eating.

The scientific research supporting mindful eating highlights its benefits beyond the realm of trendiness, presenting it as a viable method for enhancing digestive health and managing disorders like GERD. By promoting a slower, more conscious approach to eating, mindful eating aligns the body's digestive processes with the brain's satiety signals, fostering not only better physical health but also a more mindful, appreciative relationship with food. As the practice of mindful eating continues to gain traction, its potential to contribute to overall well-being and disease prevention becomes increasingly evident.

Implementing Mindful Eating Practices

The practice of mindful eating is a skill that can be cultivated over time with patience and consistent effort. Here are some steps to help you integrate mindful eating into your daily life:

Create a Mindful Eating Environment

- **Minimize Distractions**: To practice mindful eating, start by reducing distractions. Turn off the TV, put away your phone, and ensure you're seated comfortably at a table. The goal is to create a peaceful environment that allows you to focus solely on the experience of eating.

- **Professional Tip**: Nutritionists often suggest setting the table with care, even if you're dining alone, to signify that eating time is a special part of your day deserving full attention.

Engage All Your Senses

- **Sensory Appreciation**: Before you begin eating, take a moment to appreciate the presentation of your meal. Notice the colors, smell the aromas and think about the ingredients and effort that went into preparing your dish.
- **Professional Practice**: Culinary therapists recommend "seeing" your food first, then "smelling" it before you begin to eat. This practice can enhance the digestive process by signaling to your body that it's time to eat, stimulating digestive enzymes.

Eat Slowly and Savor Each Bite

- **Mindful Chewing**: Take smaller bites and chew slowly, focusing on the texture and taste of the food. This not only aids digestion by breaking down food more effectively but also enhances your enjoyment of the meal.
- **Professional Tip**: Some mindfulness coaches suggest putting down your utensils between bites as a physical reminder to slow down and assess your level of hunger and satisfaction.

Listen to Your Body's Cues

- **Hunger and Fullness**: Develop an awareness of your body's hunger signals and eat only when you feel physically hungry. Likewise, pay attention to when you feel full to avoid overeating.
- **Professional Practice**: Dietitians often teach the "hunger scale" technique, where you rate your hunger on a scale from 1 (very hungry) to 10 (overly full). Aim to start eating when you're at a 3 or 4 and stop when you're at a 6 or 7.

Practice Gratitude for Your Food

- **Gratitude Moment**: Before eating, take a moment to express gratitude for your meal. Consider the journey of the ingredients and the effort of all those who played a part in bringing the food to your table.
- **Professional Practice**: Integrating a short gratitude reflection or a moment of silence before meals can deepen the mindful eating experience, connecting you more deeply with the act of eating and the nourishment your food provides.

Reflect on Your Eating Experience

- **Post-Meal Reflection**: After eating, take a few minutes to reflect on your meal and the experience of eating mindfully. Consider what worked well and what challenges you faced.

- **Professional Tip**: Keeping a food diary with notes on your mindful eating experiences can help you identify patterns, progress, and areas for improvement.

The Emotional Gut - Mindful Eating and Emotional Health

The concept of the "emotional gut" highlights the intricate connection between our gastrointestinal health and emotional well-being. This relationship is rooted in the gut-brain axis, a complex communication network that links the emotional and cognitive centers of the brain with peripheral intestinal functions. Mindful eating plays a pivotal role in this dynamic, offering a unique approach to nurturing both emotional health and digestive wellness.

As previously touched on, our second brain has a vast network of neurons lining the gastrointestinal tract. This network communicates directly with the brain, influencing our mood, stress levels, and even our thought processes. Emotional states can trigger symptoms in the gut, and conversely, gut health can significantly impact our emotions and psychological well-being.

By fostering a mindful connection with food, individuals can engage the parasympathetic nervous system, promoting a state of calm that counteracts the stress response. This not only alleviates stress-induced digestive issues but also supports emotional balance.

Mindful eating encourages individuals to explore the emotional motivations behind their eating habits, such as eating in response to stress, sadness, or boredom. By recognizing these patterns, individuals can develop healthier coping mechanisms for emotional regulation.

By fully engaging the senses and being present during meals, mindful eating can transform eating from a routine task into a source of pleasure and satisfaction. This positive relationship with food can contribute to improved mood and overall emotional health.

The Benefits of Mindful Eating Beyond Digestion

While the positive effects of mindful eating on digestion are well-documented, its benefits extend far into other aspects of health and well-being. These broader benefits underscore mindful eating as a holistic practice that nurtures the body, mind, and spirit.

Weight Management

Mindful eating encourages eating in response to physical hunger cues rather than emotional cues or external stimuli, leading to more controlled portion sizes and reduced snacking on unhealthy foods. This approach can help in maintaining a healthy weight or losing weight naturally without restrictive dieting.

Enhanced Nutritional Choices

By slowing down and paying attention to the food we eat, mindful eating makes us more conscious of our food choices. This heightened awareness can lead to better nutritional decisions, as individuals are more likely to choose foods that are nourishing and satisfying.

Improved Mental Health

The practice of mindful eating can significantly reduce symptoms of anxiety and depression associated with eating behaviors. By promoting a non-judgmental awareness of food and eating habits, mindful eating supports a healthier self-image and body positivity.

Strengthened Mindfulness Skills

Engaging in mindful eating practices can enhance overall mindfulness skills, which can be applied to other areas of life. The principles of mindfulness learned through mindful eating —such as living in the moment, accepting experiences without judgment, and responding to signals from the body—can improve stress management, emotional regulation, and relational health.

Cultivating a Sense of Gratitude

Mindful eating often incorporates elements of gratitude, encouraging individuals to reflect on the origin of their food and the effort involved in its production. This practice fosters a deeper appreciation for food and a more profound connection to the natural world, enhancing spiritual well-being.

Mindful eating offers a comprehensive approach to health that transcends digestive wellness. By fostering a mindful, intentional relationship with food, individuals can experience a range of benefits that contribute to emotional stability, physical health, and a deeper sense of fulfillment in life.

As we delve into the profound benefits of mindful eating, it becomes clear that this practice is not just about enhancing our digestive health or managing our emotional well-being; it's a gateway to a more holistic understanding of health. Through the principles of mindfulness, we learn to listen to our bodies, honor our hunger and fullness cues, and approach our meals with gratitude and intention.

This mindful approach to eating sets a foundation for wellness that influences every aspect of our lives, including how we rest and rejuvenate. Just as mindful eating encourages us to be present and attentive to our food, it also prepares us to embrace the importance of restorative rest. The quality of our rest, much like the quality of our food, plays a critical role in our digestive health and overall vitality.

As we transition from the mindful practices at the dining table, we begin to see how these principles extend into the realm of rest, where the body continues its work of healing and rejuvenation. Thus, mindful eating becomes not just a practice in isolation but a stepping stone towards embracing a more comprehensive approach to health, one that includes the critical role of restorative rest in our digestive and overall well-being.

8
RESTORATIVE REST FOR DIGESTIVE HEALTH

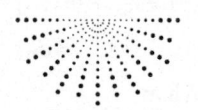

Previously we explored the intricate dance between our emotions and our gut health. We learned how feelings of stress, anxiety, and depression can stir up a whirlwind in our bellies, leading to various digestive troubles. We also delved into how we can navigate this emotional labyrinth to foster a healthier gut environment.

Now as we turn the corner, we'll trade the emotional rollercoaster for the tranquility of the night, swapping stress for slumber. We'll embark on a fascinating journey to understand how the gentle rhythm of sleep influences our gut health.

Have you ever found yourself tossing and turning at night and waking up with a troubled tummy? It's not a coincidence. Emerging research is shedding light on the intriguing link between the quality of our sleep and the health of our gut.

Through the course of this chapter, we'll explore this sleep-digestion relationship, the impact of sleep disorders on our gut, and the importance of good sleep hygiene. We'll unearth insights and strategies that will empower you to achieve restorative rest, and in turn, promote a healthier, happier gut.

So, fluff up your pillows and get cozy as we journey into the world of sleep and its profound connection with our digestive health. Let's embark on this quest for restorative rest, for the sake of our gut's health and harmony.

THE SLEEP-DIGESTION CONNECTION: EXPLORING THE IMPACT OF SLEEP ON THE GUT

Sleep and digestion, while they may seem like two independent processes, are intricately interwoven. They are both essential functions of the body and disruption in one can echo in the other, affecting overall well-being. The key to understanding this connection lies in the gut-brain axis, a complex communication network that connects our central nervous system (our brain and spinal cord) with our enteric nervous system (the nervous system within our gut).

The gut-brain axis is essentially a two-way street, it allows the brain to impact the functions of the gut, and vice versa. This intricate network is involved in a variety of physiological processes, including the regulation of sleep. Therefore, the quality and quantity of our sleep can significantly influence our gut health and, conversely, the state of our gut can impact our sleep patterns.

Evidence for this connection is provided by a study published in the World Journal of Gastroenterology. The researchers found that poor sleep quality and irregular sleep patterns could disrupt the balance of gut microbiota - the community of microorganisms living in our intestines. This disruption, known as dysbiosis, can contribute to gastrointestinal disorders such as irritable bowel syndrome (IBS) and inflammatory bowel disease (IBD) as previously discussed.

Further highlighting the impact of sleep on digestion, a study featured in the Journal of Clinical Sleep Medicine demonstrated that sleep deprivation could lead to increased gut permeability. This condition, colloquially known as 'leaky gut', can trigger inflammation and negatively impact digestion.

These findings emphasize the critical role sleep plays in maintaining optimal gut health. Ensuring we get adequate and quality sleep is not just about feeling rested, it's also about nurturing our gut microbiota and promoting our digestive health.

Understanding the Sleep-Gut Relationship

Our body operates on a circadian rhythm, or internal clock, which regulates sleep-wake cycles and also influences digestive processes. A wealth of scientific research supports this intricate connection between sleep and digestion.

A study published in BMC Gastroenterology found a significant association between sleep disturbances and digestive symptoms, including abdominal pains and acid regurgitation. This suggests that poor sleep can contribute to digestive discomfort and disorders.

On the flip side, gastrointestinal diseases also appear to be linked to sleep dysfunction. Proinflammatory cytokines, proteins that our bodies produce in response to inflammation, can disrupt sleep and are often elevated in individuals with gastrointestinal diseases. This implies that digestive health issues can lead to troubled sleep, creating a cycle that can exacerbate both sleep and digestive problems.

Moreover, studies have shown that lack of sleep can increase stress, which in turn affects the gut. When we don't get enough sleep, our hormones can become unbalanced, which can throw our digestive system off kilter. This highlights the importance of adequate sleep in maintaining hormonal balance and, consequently, gut health.

Interestingly, dietary habits also play a role in this relationship. As per emerging evidence, individuals with improper dietary habits and chronic digestive disorders often sleep less and experience lower-quality sleep. This underscores the interconnectedness of our lifestyle choices, sleep patterns, and digestive health.

Essentially, the sleep-gut relationship is a two-way street: our sleep affects our digestion, and our digestion, in turn, impacts our sleep. This underscores the importance of taking a holistic approach to health, paying attention to both our sleep habits and our diet for optimal digestive wellbeing.

Effects of Sleep Deprivation on Digestive Health

When our body doesn't get enough sleep, various physiological processes can be affected, including digestion. Sleep deprivation can lead to an array of digestive health issues, ranging from mild discomfort to serious conditions.

The intricate relationship between sleep and digestive health is a subject of growing interest within the medical and scientific communities. The effects of sleep deprivation on the gastrointestinal system are multifaceted, impacting everything from hormone regulation to the gut microbiome. This exploration delves into the physiological mechanisms affected by lack of sleep and how they relate to digestive health, supported by empirical evidence and studies.

Hormonal Imbalance and Inflammation

One of the primary ways in which sleep deprivation affects digestion is through the dysregulation of stress hormones, notably cortisol. Cortisol, often referred to as the "stress hormone," plays a critical role in various bodily functions, including metabolism and the inflammatory response. Under normal circumstances, cortisol levels follow a diurnal rhythm, peaking in the morning and tapering off at night. However, insufficient sleep can disrupt this rhythm, leading to elevated cortisol levels.

Elevated cortisol can have a pro-inflammatory effect on the body, which is detrimental to digestive health. Chronic inflammation can compromise the integrity of the gastrointestinal lining, making it more susceptible to irritation and increasing the risk of conditions such as gastritis, indigestion, and acid reflux. The correlation between disrupted sleep patterns and increased inflammation underscores the importance of restorative sleep for maintaining the mucosal barrier, a crucial defense mechanism of the digestive tract.

Gastroesophageal Reflux Disease (GERD) and Sleep Deprivation

The link between sleep deprivation and gastroesophageal

reflux disease (GERD) is particularly well-documented. GERD is characterized by the backward flow of stomach acid into the esophagus, leading to symptoms such as heartburn and acid regurgitation. A pivotal study published in the World Journal of Gastroenterology found that individuals experiencing inadequate sleep were significantly more likely to suffer from GERD compared to those with sufficient sleep. This association suggests that sleep quality and duration can directly influence the severity and frequency of acid reflux episodes.

Several mechanisms may underlie this relationship. For instance, sleep deprivation can alter the pressure gradient in the lower esophageal sphincter (LES), the valve that prevents stomach acid from entering the esophagus. Additionally, lack of sleep can exacerbate the perception of pain, making GERD symptoms feel more severe. It also impacts the rate at which the stomach empties, with delayed gastric emptying potentially worsening reflux symptoms.

Broader Implications for Digestive Health

Beyond GERD, sleep deprivation has broader implications for digestive health. It can affect appetite regulation by altering the levels of hunger hormones ghrelin and leptin, potentially leading to overeating or unhealthy eating habits that further compromise digestive health. Furthermore, the disruption of the gut microbiome—a critical component of gastrointestinal health—has been observed in the context of sleep deprivation. An imbalanced gut microbiota can contribute to a range of digestive issues, from bloating and gas to more serious conditions like inflammatory bowel disease (IBD).

the effects of sleep deprivation on digestive health are profound and multifaceted, impacting everything from hormone regulation and inflammatory responses to the microbiome and gastric motility. These insights underscore the necessity of prioritizing sleep as a key component of digestive health and overall well-being. By addressing sleep issues, individuals can take a crucial step towards mitigating the risk of digestive disorders and enhancing their quality of life.

The Role of Quality Sleep in Digestive Wellness

Quality sleep is not just about resting after a long day, it's a fundamental aspect of maintaining and promoting digestive health. When we sleep, our bodies are hard at work, processing the food consumed during the day and breaking it down to extract vital nutrients. This rest and repair state enhances digestion and absorption efficiency. A study published in the American Journal of Physiology found that sleep can influence the secretion of digestive enzymes, thereby improving digestion efficiency.

Additionally, good quality sleep contributes significantly to the health of our gut microbiome, a collection of beneficial bacteria in our digestive system. The gut microbiome plays a crucial role in our overall health, including digestion, immune function, and even mental health. A study in Frontiers in Psychiatry highlighted the role of sleep in regulating the gut microbiome, indicating that sleep deprivation can lead to an imbalance in this delicate ecosystem, known as dysbiosis, which can contribute to various health issues.

Moreover, quality sleep can help in avoiding various

gastrointestinal issues. Research published in the World Journal of Gastroenterology found that sleep deprivation is associated with an increased risk of gastroesophageal reflux disease (GERD) and irritable bowel syndrome (IBS). Thus, ensuring quality sleep can help prevent such conditions.

Quality sleep can help reduce inflammation in the body, including within the digestive system. Inflammatory responses can often lead to digestive discomfort and disorders. A study in the Journal of Experimental Medicine found that sleep can modulate inflammatory responses, thereby promoting better digestive health.

In summary, here are the key roles of quality sleep in promoting digestive wellness:

- Enhances digestion and absorption of nutrients.
- Regulates the gut microbiome, contributing to overall health.
- It helps prevent various gastrointestinal issues such as GERD and IBS.
- Reduces inflammation in the body, promoting better digestive health.

Circadian Rhythms and Digestive Health

The human body operates on a 24-hour internal clock, also known as the circadian rhythm. This biological rhythm influences a wide range of physiological processes, including digestion. Just as we have a sleep-wake cycle, our digestive system follows a pattern too, working in sync with our circadian rhythm.

Primarily, circadian rhythms regulate the timing of food intake and digestion. Our bodies are designed to consume food during the day and rest at night, allowing the digestive system time to process nutrients and recover. A study in the Journal of Biological Rhythms found that disruptions to these rhythms, such as eating late at night, can impair digestion and contribute to metabolic disorders.

Additionally, circadian rhythms influence the release of digestive enzymes and the rate of gastric emptying. This means our bodies are more equipped to digest and absorb food at certain times of the day. Research published in the American Journal of Physiology demonstrates that our bodies secrete more digestive enzymes during the day, aligning with typical meal times.

The gut microbiome, a vital player in our digestive health, is also under the influence of the circadian rhythm. The composition and function of these bacteria change throughout the day, impacting nutrient processing and overall gut health. A study in Cell Reports highlighted the link between disrupted circadian rhythms and dysbiosis of the gut microbiome, which can lead to digestive issues.

Circadian rhythms can affect gastrointestinal motility, the movement of food through the digestive tract. Studies have found that disruptions in circadian rhythms may contribute to conditions like Irritable Bowel Syndrome (IBS) and Gastroesophageal Reflux Disease (GERD).

The circadian rhythms play a crucial role in:

- Regulating the timing of food intake and digestion.

- Influencing the release of digestive enzymes and the rate of gastric emptying.
- Modulating the gut microbiome's composition and function.
- This affects gastrointestinal motility and thus the movement of food through the digestive tract.

The Role of Circadian Rhythm in Body Temperature

The circadian rhythm influences the body's temperature regulation, causing a natural decline in core body temperature in the evening, signaling that it's time to sleep. This temperature drop is facilitated by the dilation of blood vessels in the skin, particularly in the hands and feet, allowing heat to escape from the body's core and lower the overall temperature. This process is known as vasodilation.

The Thermoregulatory Process

- **Melatonin and Temperature Drop**: The release of melatonin, often referred to as the "sleep hormone," is closely linked to this cooling process. As the environment darkens, the pineal gland in the brain secretes melatonin, which not only induces drowsiness but also helps lower the body's core temperature. This cooling effect is crucial for falling asleep and progressing through the sleep cycles efficiently.
- **Optimal Sleep Temperature**: Research indicates that the optimal room temperature for sleep is

between 60 to 67 degrees Fahrenheit (about 15.6 to 19.4 degrees Celsius). This range supports the body's natural temperature drop and can help facilitate the onset of sleep as well as its duration and quality.

Implications of Disrupted Temperature Regulation

Failure to achieve this drop in body temperature can lead to difficulties in falling asleep and staying asleep. Conditions that disrupt the body's ability to regulate temperature, such as hyperthyroidism, menopause, or certain sleep disorders, can interfere with sleep quality. Moreover, environments that are too warm or too cold can hinder the body's natural temperature adjustments, leading to fragmented sleep and decreased sleep efficiency.

Practical Applications for Enhancing Sleep Quality

Understanding the relationship between body temperature and sleep has practical applications for improving sleep hygiene:

- **Cool Environment**: Keeping the bedroom at a cooler temperature can aid the body's natural cooling process.
- **Warm Baths or Showers**: Taking a warm bath or shower 1-2 hours before bedtime can increase the body's surface temperature temporarily. Afterward, the rapid cool-down period mimetically aids the

natural drop in body temperature, promoting drowsiness.
- **Lightweight Bedding and Clothing**: Using breathable, lightweight bedding and sleepwear can facilitate heat loss and maintain a comfortable sleep environment.

Practical Tips for Enhancing Sleep for Better Digestion

Good sleep is a cornerstone of health. Yet, many of us struggle to get enough sleep and wake up feeling rested. The good news is that it doesn't have to be this way. By following some simple tips recommended by professionals, we can improve our sleep quality, and consequently, our digestion and overall well-being.

Professionals in the fields of sleep research and gastroenterology have long recognized the connection between good sleep and healthy digestion. Here's what they recommend:

- **Regular Sleep Schedule:** Try to go to bed and wake up at the same time every day, including on weekends. This consistency reinforces your body's sleep-wake cycle and can help promote better sleep.
- **Conducive Environment:** Make your bedroom quiet, dark, and cool for optimal sleep conditions. Consider using room-darkening shades or a fan to create a more comfortable sleeping environment.
- **Mindful of Naps:** If you must nap, aim for short naps during mid-afternoon. Extended napping or napping late in the day can disrupt your sleep.

- **Regular Exercise:** Regular physical activity can help you fall asleep faster and enjoy deeper sleep.
- **Manage Stress:** Before you go to bed, take steps to manage stress and worries. This can make it easier to get to sleep and stay asleep.
- **Avoid Heavy Evening Meals:** Eating heavy meals close to bedtime can lead to discomfort and indigestion, making it harder to sleep.
- **Stay Hydrated but Be Mindful:** It's important to stay hydrated, but try to avoid drinking large amounts of liquids close to bedtime to minimize nighttime trips to the bathroom.

SLEEP HYGIENE FOR GUT HARMONY: BEST PRACTICES FOR RESTFUL SLEEP

The importance of sleep on our overall health is undeniable, but its impact on our gut health is an area that's gaining increasing attention. As we've mentioned before, sleep and digestion are interconnected and mediated by the gut-brain axis. This means that sleep quality and duration can have a profound effect on our gut health, and vice versa. Therefore, optimizing sleep hygiene - the behaviors and habits that can enhance sleep quality - is crucial for promoting gut health.

According to the National Sleep Foundation, several practices can improve sleep hygiene. Maintaining a consistent sleep schedule, for example, can regulate your body's internal clock and help you fall asleep and wake up more easily. This includes going to bed at the same time each night and waking up at the same time each morning, even on weekends.

Creating a sleep-friendly environment is another key aspect of sleep hygiene. This could involve ensuring your bedroom is dark, quiet, and cool, and investing in a comfortable mattress and pillows. It might also mean making your bedroom a screen-free zone, as electronic devices emit light that can interfere with your body's production of melatonin, a hormone that regulates sleep. Let us delve into some of these further.

Heavy Meals

Eating heavy or large meals close to bedtime can cause discomfort and indigestion, making it harder to fall asleep. The digestive process requires significant energy and can lead to physical discomfort, as well as increased metabolism and body temperature, all of which are counterproductive to the body's natural cooling down process necessary for sleep initiation.

Caffeine and Alcohol

Caffeine is a well-known stimulant found in coffee, tea, chocolate, and many sodas and energy drinks. Its consumption can delay the body's internal clock, reduce total sleep time, and impair sleep quality, particularly if consumed in the late afternoon or evening. Alcohol, while initially sedative, can significantly disrupt the sleep cycle, leading to fragmented sleep patterns and reducing the time spent in REM sleep, which is crucial for cognitive functions such as memory and learning.

Intense Exercise

While regular exercise is beneficial for sleep, engaging in intense physical activities close to bedtime can have the opposite effect. High-energy workouts can increase heart rate and body temperature, energizing the body and mind at a time when they should be winding down. However, this doesn't mean all physical activity should be avoided; gentle, relaxing exercises like yoga or stretching can promote sleep.

Screen Time

The blue light emitted by screens from smartphones, tablets, computers, and televisions can interfere with the production of melatonin, the hormone responsible for regulating sleep-wake cycles. Exposure to blue light in the evening can trick the brain into thinking it's still daytime, thus delaying sleepiness and reducing the quality of sleep. The study published in the Journal of Sleep Medicine Reviews underscores the association between excessive screen time before bed and poor sleep quality, emphasizing the impact of blue light exposure on sleep.

By adhering to good sleep hygiene practices, we can foster better sleep quality and duration, which in turn can promote gut harmony and overall health.

ADDRESSING SLEEP DISORDERS: APPROACHES TO MANAGING SLEEP ISSUES FOR DIGESTIVE BENEFITS

Sleep issues are not to be taken lightly. Persistent sleep disturbances can impact various aspects of our health, including our gut health. Therefore, addressing these issues is not only crucial for overall well-being but also for maintaining a healthy digestive system.

One effective approach to managing sleep disorders is Cognitive Behavioral Therapy for Insomnia (CBT-I). This structured program aids in identifying and altering thoughts and behaviors that exacerbate sleep problems. A study published in the Journal of Sleep Research supports the effectiveness of this approach, revealing that CBT-I not only improved sleep disorders but also alleviated digestive symptoms in individuals with sleep disturbances.

However, self-management of sleep issues might not always be sufficient. Persistent sleep problems may be a sign of underlying conditions that require professional intervention. Therefore, it is essential to consult with a healthcare professional if you're struggling with sleep issues. They can help identify the root cause of the problem and guide you toward appropriate treatments.

Understanding the connection between sleep quality and digestive health, and implementing best sleep practices, is key to achieving gut harmony. A good night's sleep can leave you feeling more refreshed and balanced so sleep tight for a healthy gut!

Sleep Disorders

Sleep disorders are conditions that frequently impact your ability to get enough quality sleep. The most common types of sleep disorders include:

Insomnia

Insomnia is the most common sleep disorder. It involves difficulty falling asleep, staying asleep, or both. People with insomnia often wake up feeling tired or don't feel refreshed when they wake up. This disorder can be acute (short-term) or chronic (long-term), with the latter being diagnosed when the symptoms occur at least three nights per week for three months or more.

Sleep Apnea

Sleep apnea is a serious sleep disorder where breathing repeatedly stops and starts during sleep. There are two main types: Obstructive Sleep Apnea (OSA), the more common form that occurs when throat muscles relax, and Central Sleep Apnea (CSA), that occurs when your brain doesn't send proper signals to the muscles that control breathing. This disorder can lead to poor quality sleep and excessive daytime fatigue.

Restless Legs Syndrome (RLS)

Restless Legs Syndrome is a neurological disorder characterized by an uncontrollable urge to move your legs, usually due to discomfort. These sensations are often described as crawling, creeping, pulling, or painful. The symptoms typically occur or worsen during periods of rest or inactivity, particularly in the evening or at night when sitting or lying down, leading to disturbed sleep and daytime fatigue.

Narcolepsy

Narcolepsy is a chronic sleep disorder characterized by overwhelming daytime drowsiness and sudden attacks of sleep. People with narcolepsy often find it difficult to stay awake for long periods, regardless of the circumstances. It also includes features of dreaming, like rapid eye movement (REM) sleep, that occur while you're awake. It's often associated with sudden loss of muscle tone (cataplexy), which leads to weakness and loss of muscle control.

Effects of Sleep Disorders

Sleep disorders can have a significant impact on your health. Here are some potential complications:

- **Mental Health Disorders**: Sleep disorders can contribute to problems such as depression, anxiety, and cognitive dysfunction.
- **Immune Function**: Chronic sleep loss can affect your immune system, making you more susceptible to infections.

- **Cardiovascular Disease**: Sleep disorders have been linked with increased risk of heart disease, high blood pressure, and stroke.
- **Obesity and Other Health Problems**: Lack of sleep can lead to weight gain and increase the risk of diabetes and other health problems.
- **Performance Issues**: Sleep disorders can result in decreased productivity, concentration, and quality of life.

Approaches to Manage Sleep Disorders

Several strategies can be effective in managing sleep disorders:

- **Cognitive Behavioral Therapy for Insomnia (CBT-I)**: This structured program helps you identify and replace thoughts and behaviors that worsen sleep problems. It's been shown to improve sleep disorders and digestive symptoms effectively.
- **Medication**: In some cases, prescription or over-the-counter medication may be recommended by your healthcare provider.
- **Lifestyle Changes**: Regular exercise, a healthy diet, a consistent sleep schedule, and reducing caffeine and alcohol can improve sleep.
- **Relaxation Techniques**: Techniques such as deep breathing, meditation, and yoga can help you relax before bed and improve sleep quality.

- **Consultation with a Healthcare Professional**: If you're experiencing persistent sleep issues, a professional can identify underlying issues and guide you toward appropriate treatments.

Understanding and addressing sleep disorders is a vital part of maintaining our overall health. As we've explored, conditions like insomnia, sleep apnea, restless legs syndrome, and narcolepsy can significantly impact our sleep quality and, consequently, our well-being. But the journey to optimal health doesn't stop at ensuring we're getting quality sleep. Sleep is just one piece of the complex health puzzle.

The next crucial factor we need to consider is the balance of our microbiome. To truly thrive, we need to nurture and balance the billions of bacteria that live in our bodies, specifically in our gut. This balance plays an integral role in everything from our digestion to our mood to our immune system. So, let's move forward and explore how we can optimize our microbiome for better health and vitality.

9
BALANCING THE MICROBIOME

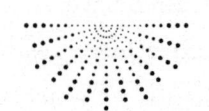

Imagine a bustling city, alive with activity at every corner. The streets are filled with individuals, each with a unique purpose and function, collectively contributing to the harmony and prosperity of their thriving metropolis. Now, picture this scene not in a sprawling urban landscape, but within the confines of your own body. This is the world of your microbiome, a complex and fascinating universe teeming with trillions of microbes. Their mission? To maintain your health and keep your systems in perfect balance.

But what happens when this balance is disrupted, and how do we reclaim control? Let us delve into an extraordinary tale of microbiome recovery, where restoring balance leads to survival and a revitalized life full of health and vitality. Ready to embark on this adventure? then let's get to it.

MICROBIOME ANALYSIS: UNDERSTANDING THE STATE OF YOUR GUT FLORA

As we journeyed through the previous chapters, we've gained an understanding of the microbiome - the complex community of trillions of microbes residing primarily in our gut, so let us refresh our memory before moving on. The human microbiome, particularly the gut microbiome, consists of trillions of microorganisms, including bacteria, viruses, fungi, and protozoa.

This complex community resides mainly in the gastrointestinal tract and has a profound impact on human physiology, health, and disease. The microbiome aids in digestion, synthesizes essential vitamins, and plays a critical role in training and regulating the immune system. As we've learned, this community plays a crucial role in maintaining our health by aiding digestion, producing vital vitamins, and training our immune system.

The Intricacies of Gut Flora Balance

The gut flora is a dynamic and diverse ecosystem, with a delicate balance between various microorganisms. This balance is crucial for gut health and overall well-being. Dysbiosis, or the imbalance of gut flora, is associated with a wide range of health issues, including digestive disorders like irritable bowel syndrome (IBS) and inflammatory bowel diseases (IBD), as well as systemic conditions such as obesity, diabetes, and even mental health disorders (Carding, Verbeke, Vipond, Corfe, & Owen, 2015).

A pivotal study by Turnbaugh et al. (2009) demonstrated a significant association between gut flora composition and obesity in mice. The researchers found that obese mice had a higher ratio of Firmicutes to Bacteroidetes, two major bacterial phyla in the gut, compared to their lean counterparts. This altered ratio was associated with increased energy harvest from the diet, contributing to obesity.

The Human Microbiome Project has revolutionized our understanding of the human microbiome. One of the key findings is that a "healthy" microbiome is not characterized by the presence of specific microbial species but rather by its genetic diversity and the functional capabilities of its microbial community. This functional resilience is crucial for maintaining health and responding to environmental stresses (Human Microbiome Project Consortium, 2012).

Diversity within the gut microbiome is a hallmark of good health. A diverse microbiome is more capable of resisting disturbances, whether from diet, lifestyle, or antibiotic use and is associated with a lower risk of chronic diseases. The richness of microbial species ensures a wide range of metabolic capabilities, from breaking down dietary fibers to synthesizing vitamins and essential amino acids (Lozupone et al., 2012).

Microbiome Analysis Techniques

To further elucidate the methodologies for microbiome analysis, let's delve into the specifics of each technique, highlighting their applications, advantages, and limitations. These methodologies have significantly advanced our understanding of the gut microbiome, providing insights into its composition, function, and role in health and disease.

16S rRNA Sequencing

16S rRNA sequencing targets the 16S ribosomal RNA gene, a component of the prokaryotic ribosome that is highly conserved among bacterial species. However, certain regions within the gene exhibit variability that can be exploited for bacterial identification and classification.

Advantages

- **Specificity:** The variability in the 16S rRNA gene allows for the differentiation between closely related bacterial species.
- **Cost-Effectiveness:** It is less expensive than whole-genome sequencing methods, making it accessible for large-scale studies.

Limitations

- **Resolution:** While effective at identifying bacteria at the genus level, it may not always provide species-level resolution.
- **Bacterial Focus:** It exclusively identifies bacteria, overlooking other components of the microbiome such as fungi, viruses, and archaea.

Metagenomic Sequencing

Metagenomic sequencing involves the direct sequencing of all the genetic material present in an environmental sample, providing a comprehensive overview of the microbial community's genetic diversity and functional potential.

Advantages

- **Comprehensive Analysis:** It captures the entire genomic content of microbial communities, including bacteria, viruses, fungi, and archaea.
- **Functional Insights:** Beyond identifying microbes, it allows for the prediction of their functional capabilities based on the presence of specific genes.

Limitations

- **Complexity and Cost:** The analysis of metagenomic data is complex and resource-intensive, requiring sophisticated bioinformatics tools and expertise.
- **Data Overload:** The vast amount of data generated can be challenging to manage and interpret.

Metatranscriptomics

Metatranscriptomics goes a step further by sequencing the RNA in a sample, providing insights into the active metabolic processes and functional state of the microbial community at the time of sampling.

Advantages

- **Dynamic Insights:** It reveals which genes are being actively transcribed, offering a snapshot of the microbiome's functional activity.
- **Functional Validation:** Complements metagenomic data by confirming which genes are actively contributing to the microbiome's functional output.

Limitations

- **Technical Challenges:** RNA is less stable than DNA, making sample processing and RNA extraction more challenging.
- **Interpretation Complexity:** The data analysis requires advanced bioinformatics approaches to link gene expression patterns to microbial functions and processes.

Deciphering the Data

Interpreting the data from microbiome analyses can be a complex task due to its richness and complexity. However, some key points can help you understand your results:

- **Diversity:** A diverse gut microbiota is generally considered healthy. It is usually measured in two ways: richness (the number of different types of bacteria) and evenness (how evenly distributed these bacteria are) (Shannon et al., 2003).

- **Abundance of Key Taxa:** Certain types of bacteria have been associated with specific health outcomes. For example, a high abundance of Firmicutes relative to Bacteroidetes has been linked to obesity (Ley et al., 2006).
- **Functional Potential:** Metagenomic and metatranscriptomic analyses can provide insights into the potential functions of your gut microbiota, such as the production of short-chain fatty acids, which are beneficial for gut health (Den Besten et al., 2013).

Case Studies of Microbiome Recovery

This complex ecosystem plays a crucial role in our overall health, influencing everything from digestion to the immune response, and even our mood. However, factors such as diet, lifestyle, and medication, particularly antibiotics, can disrupt this delicate balance.

When dysbiosis occurs, it can have far-reaching effects on our health, contributing to conditions such as obesity, diabetes, and even mental health disorders. But the good news is, that our microbiome has an incredible capacity to recover, given the right support.

The following case studies illustrate the journey of three individuals who faced significant health challenges related to their gut microbiome. Through personalized interventions, they were able to restore balance to their gut, highlighting the resilience of the microbiome and its central role in our health. You'll see how changes in diet, including the role of red meat, the use of probiotics, and innovative medical procedures like Fecal Microbiota Transplantation (FMT) can support microbiome recovery. Let's dive into their stories.

Case Study 1: Antibiotic-Induced Dysbiosis Recovery

John, a 35-year-old man, experienced gut microbiome dysbiosis after a course of broad-spectrum antibiotics for a respiratory infection. He suffered from bloating, irregular bowel movements, and fatigue. After a comprehensive stool analysis, it was confirmed that his gut microbiome diversity was significantly reduced.

John's recovery plan included a high-fiber diet rich in fruits, vegetables, legumes, and whole grains to promote the growth of beneficial bacteria. He also took a specific probiotic supplement (Lactobacillus and Bifidobacterium strains) and prebiotics. After six months, a follow-up microbiome analysis showed a remarkable improvement in the diversity and balance of his gut flora. His symptoms also significantly improved.

Case Study 2: Dietary Intervention for Gut Health

Sarah, a 50-year-old woman, was dealing with obesity and type-2 diabetes. Her gut microbiome analysis showed an overabundance of Firmicutes and lack of Bacteroidetes, a pattern often associated with obesity.

Sarah's recovery plan involved a Mediterranean diet, which is known for its potential to alter gut microbiota favorably. She was encouraged to consume more plant-based foods, lean proteins, and healthy fats while reducing processed foods and sugars. After a year of dietary changes, her gut microbiota showed an increased proportion of Bacteroidetes and reduced Firmicutes. She also lost weight and had improved glycemic control.

Case Study 3: Fecal Microbiota Transplantation (FMT)

George, a 65-year-old man, suffered from recurrent Clostridioides difficile infection, a condition linked with severe gut microbiome imbalance. When conventional treatments failed, George underwent Fecal Microbiota Transplantation (FMT). Healthy donor fecal matter was transplanted into George's gut to re-establish a balanced microbiota.

Post-FMT, George's symptoms significantly improved, with no recurrences of C. difficile infection. Follow-up microbiome analysis showed a diverse and balanced gut microbiota, resembling the healthy donor's profile.

These case studies illustrate how personalized dietary interventions, probiotics, and even innovative procedures like FMT can help in microbiome recovery. However, it's essential to remember that each individual's microbiome is unique, and what works for one may not work for another. Always consult with healthcare professionals for personalized advice.

These case studies collectively highlight the critical role of the gut microbiome in overall health and the potential of personalized interventions—including diet modifications, probiotic and prebiotic supplementation, and medical procedures like FMT—to restore microbiome health. They also emphasize the need for healthcare professionals' guidance in developing tailored treatment plans, considering the unique nature of each individual's microbiome.

Fine-Tuning Your Microbiome Strategy

Before you dive into any gut health strategies, it's essential to understand the results of your microbiome analysis. This analysis, often conducted through a stool sample test, provides a snapshot of the bacteria residing in your gut. It can reveal the diversity of your gut flora, the presence of beneficial or harmful bacteria, and potential imbalances that could impact your health.

Personalized Diet Strategies

Your diet is one of the most impactful ways to modify your gut microbiome. The foods you eat can either foster a diverse and healthy gut flora or contribute to dysbiosis. Based on your microbiome analysis, consider the following tips:

- **Increase Fiber Intake**: Foods rich in dietary fiber like fruits, vegetables, legumes, and whole grains feed your gut bacteria and help them thrive.
- **Consider Fermented Foods**: These foods, such as yogurt, kefir, sauerkraut, and kimchi, contain probiotics that can boost the diversity of your gut flora.
- **Balance Protein Sources**: While protein is essential, the source matters. Plant-based proteins are linked with a healthier gut microbiome. Remember, red

meat can be part of a balanced diet, but it's best consumed in moderation due to its potential impact on gut microbiota.

Lifestyle Modifications

Beyond diet, your lifestyle can significantly influence your gut health.

- **Regular Exercise**: Engaging in regular physical activity can diversify your gut microbiota and strengthen your gut barrier function.
- **Adequate Sleep**: Poor sleep can disturb your gut flora. Ensure you're getting enough quality sleep.
- **Stress Management**: High-stress levels can upset your gut balance. Techniques such as meditation, yoga, or mindfulness can help manage stress levels, promoting a healthier gut.

Medical Interventions

In some cases, medical interventions might be necessary, especially if you're dealing with persistent gut health issues.

- **Probiotic Supplementation**: Depending on your microbiome analysis, specific probiotic strains might be beneficial. Always consult a healthcare provider before starting any new supplement regimen.

- **Fecal Microbiota Transplantation (FMT)**: For serious conditions like recurrent Clostridioides difficile infection, FMT might be considere.

DIETARY INTERVENTIONS: ADJUSTING YOUR DIET TO REBALANCE THE MICROBIOME

The food we eat plays a crucial role in shaping the microbiota residing in our gut. By making strategic dietary changes, we can influence the diversity and health of our gut flora.

Diverse Plant-Based Foods

A diet rich in a variety of plant-based foods is a cornerstone of a healthy gut microbiome. Here's why:

- **Diversity**: Eating a wide range of plant-based foods can lead to a more diverse gut microbiome, which is associated with better health. Different types of bacteria thrive on different types of fiber, so by eating a diverse diet, you provide a wider range of nutrients for your gut bacteria.
- **Fiber**: Plant-based foods are packed with dietary fiber, which our bodies can't digest, but our gut bacteria can. As they ferment the fiber, they produce short-chain fatty acids, which have numerous health benefits, including reducing inflammation and promoting gut health.
- **Polyphenols**: These are plant compounds with antioxidant properties that are found in fruits,

vegetables, legumes, and whole grains. They can help to reduce inflammation and are also beneficial to the gut microbiome.

Examples of diverse plant-based foods include various fruits and vegetables, legumes like lentils and chickpeas, and whole grains such as brown rice, oats, and quinoa.

Limit Processed Foods

In the pursuit of a healthy lifestyle, one of the first pieces of advice you'll often hear is to limit the intake of processed foods. But why is this so crucial? Processed foods can negatively impact our gut health in several ways, leading to a variety of health issues.

Processed foods often contain additives, preservatives, artificial colors, and flavors that can disrupt the balance of our gut microbiota – the collection of beneficial bacteria residing in our digestive system. These substances can diminish the diversity of our gut bacteria, which is key to a healthy digestion and overall well-being.

Moreover, processed foods are typically high in unhealthy fats, sugars, and salt, and low in fiber, which is essential for a healthy gut. Overconsumption can lead to inflammation, obesity, heart disease, and other health problems.

Processed foods can be detrimental to our gut health for several reasons:

- **High in Sugar**: Many processed foods are high in sugars, which can lead to an overgrowth of certain

types of bacteria and yeasts in the gut that thrive on sugar, potentially crowding out beneficial bacteria.
- **Saturated Fats**: Processed foods often contain unhealthy fats, which can promote inflammation and negatively impact the balance of gut bacteria.
- **Artificial Additives**: Many processed foods contain additives, such as emulsifiers and artificial sweeteners, that can disrupt the gut microbiome. Some research suggests that these additives may even promote inflammation and obesity.
- **Low in Fiber**: Processed foods are often low in fiber, the primary food source for your gut bacteria. A lack of dietary fiber can lead to a less diverse gut microbiome.

Striving to minimize processed food intake is a commendable step towards improved health. Aiming for whole, fresh foods at every opportunity is a practical and beneficial approach. When buying packaged foods, prefer products with a succinct list of ingredients, and avoid those containing ingredients that are unfamiliar or difficult to pronounce.

Furthermore, taking the initiative to research the ingredients found in processed foods can be enlightening. Understanding the potential toxicity and harmful impact of certain ingredients can serve as a powerful deterrent against future consumption. By making these conscious choices, you are not only safeguarding your health but also empowering yourself with knowledge.

Prebiotic-Rich Foods

Prebiotics are a type of dietary fiber that serves as food for the beneficial bacteria in your gut. They're a crucial part of maintaining a healthy microbiome. Here's how:

- **Feeding Beneficial Bacteria**: Prebiotics feed your gut's good bacteria, helping them thrive and multiply. This can improve your overall gut health and boost your immune system.
- **Improving Digestive Health**: By stimulating the growth and activity of beneficial gut bacteria, prebiotics help to improve digestion and nutrient absorption.
- **Supporting Overall Health**: Some research suggests that prebiotics may help to reduce inflammation, lower cholesterol levels, and improve blood sugar control.

Prebiotic-rich foods include garlic, onions, bananas, and oats, but also others like asparagus, leeks, and whole wheat products.

Hydrate

Staying hydrated is important for your overall health, and it plays a key role in maintaining a healthy gut as well.

- **Maintaining Mucosal Lining**: Water helps to maintain the mucosal lining of the intestines - an

important barrier that helps to protect your body from harmful substances while allowing nutrients to be absorbed.
- **Aiding Digestion**: Water aids in digestion by helping to break down food and absorb nutrients. It also helps to soften stool, preventing constipation.
- **Supporting Beneficial Bacteria**: Staying hydrated may also help to support the balance and growth of beneficial gut bacteria.

As a general guideline, aim to drink at least 8 glasses of water a day, but remember that individual needs can vary based on factors like age, activity level, and climate.

Probiotics

Probiotics are live bacteria and yeasts that are good for our health, especially the digestive system. Here's how to integrate them into your lifestyle:

Probiotic-Rich Foods

Fermented foods like yogurt, kefir, sauerkraut, and kimchi are natural sources of probiotics. Incorporating these into your diet can help diversify your gut flora.

Probiotic Supplements

These can be an effective way to introduce specific strains of beneficial bacteria into your gut. However, it's crucial to consult with a healthcare provider, as the effectiveness of probiotics can vary based on the strain and individual's health needs.

Strain Specificity

Different probiotic strains offer different health benefits, so it's important to choose the right one based on your health needs. For example, Lactobacillus species are often used for their ability to promote a healthy gut and immune system.

Quality Matters

Not all probiotics are created equal. When selecting a probiotic supplement, look for products that have been third-party tested for quality and potency.

Incorporating probiotics into your lifestyle, whether through diet or supplementation, can support a healthy and diverse gut microbiome. However, they are not a cure-all and should be part of an overall healthy lifestyle that includes a balanced diet, regular exercise, and good sleep habits.

Just as diet plays a crucial role in shaping our gut microbiome, so too do lifestyle factors. While we've focused on the importance of nutrition for gut health, it's only one piece of the puzzle. An integrative approach that encompasses the whole body can create an environment that allows your gut microbiome to thrive. This is where holistic practices come into play.

As we move into the final chapter, we'll explore how incorporating holistic practices, such as mindfulness, exercise, and restorative sleep, can support your gut health and enhance your overall well-being. Ultimately, the journey to a healthier gut is not just about what you eat, but also about how you live. So, let's turn the page and dive into these holistic practices that can bolster the health of your gut microbiome and, by extension, your overall health.

10
INTEGRATING HOLISTIC PRACTICES

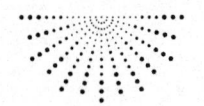

Have you ever heard the story of Sarah, a high-powered corporate lawyer from New York? For years, she wrestled with persistent digestive issues. She woke up to stomach pains in the morning, dealt with bloating and discomfort after every meal, and often had to cancel social events due to her unpredictable gut. She tried everything from trendy diets to heavy-duty medications, but nothing seemed to make a lasting difference. That was until she discovered the world of holistic practices. Intrigued, she decided to give it a shot.

Sarah began attending yoga classes three times a week, took up meditation every morning, and made it a priority to ensure she was getting quality sleep every night. She started to notice improvements within a couple of weeks - her stomach was less bloated, and the morning stomach pains were no longer a daily occurrence. After a few months, she felt an energy and vitality she hadn't felt in years. Her digestion improved, her sleep was more restful, and she found herself better able to handle the stresses of her demanding job. This transformation in Sarah's health is a testament to the power of holistic practices in not just improving gut health, but overall well-being too.

In this chapter, we will delve deeper into the world of holistic practices and their influence on gut health. We'll explore how integrating these practices into your lifestyle can complement your diet and further boost your gut health. From the calming effects of mindfulness to the restorative power of quality sleep and the invigorating influence of regular exercise, these practices can have profound effects on your well-being.

We'll guide you through different techniques and tools you can incorporate into your life, creating a holistic routine that not only supports your gut health but also contributes to your overall wellness. Remember Sarah's story - a shift in lifestyle can lead to a dramatic transformation in gut health. And who knows? Your transformation might be just around the corner. Let's journey together into the world of holistic practices and their impact on gut health.

BEYOND DIET AND EXERCISE: EXPLORING ADDITIONAL PRACTICES

Diet and exercise indisputably form the bedrock of good health, but they're not the only pieces of the puzzle. In our pursuit of holistic well-being, it's essential to look beyond just these two factors. Here, we delve into additional practices that complement diet and exercise.

Mindful Eating

Mindful eating is a practice that encourages a heightened awareness of physical and emotional sensations while eating. It involves paying full attention to the process of eating, including recognizing your body's hunger and satiety cues. Research has indicated that mindful eating can help improve digestion, reduce overeating, and foster a healthier relationship with food, which are all crucial for maintaining gut health.

For instance, a clinical review has demonstrated the connection between Neurogastrointestinal physiology and stress, suggesting that mindful eating can be used to improve digestion. Other research has shown that mindfulness may reduce digestive symptoms in people, offering potential benefits for overall health.

Hydration

Adequate hydration is essential for digestive health and nutrient absorption. Water plays a critical role in maintaining the lining of the intestines, promoting their optimal function. Studies have shown that drinking water can significantly shape the human gut microbiome. Thus, maintaining good hydration can contribute to a healthier gut.

Low-water drinkers also showed gut microbiota differences compared with high-water drinkers, indicating that adequate hydration is key to a balanced gut microbiome. Another study reaffirmed that adequate hydration can affect digestion, inflammation, and metabolism. here are some examples of the different forms your water can come in:

Tap Water

Tap water, the most accessible form of water is treated to remove contaminants and pathogens, making it safe to drink in most parts of the world. It contains minerals that can be beneficial for health, including magnesium and calcium, which are essential for bone health and may also play a role in maintaining a healthy gut microbiome.

However, the quality of tap water can vary depending on the location and the effectiveness of local water treatment processes. This form of water has been known to contain a range of contaminants such as heavy metals and synthetic chemicals.

Mineral Water

Mineral water is sourced from underground reservoirs and springs, naturally rich in minerals like calcium, magnesium, and potassium. These minerals can contribute to the electrolyte balance in the body and support digestion by promoting the secretion of digestive juices and enzymes. Drinking mineral water could also potentially offer a slight edge in promoting a healthy gut microbiome by introducing a variety of minerals that support overall gut health.

Distilled Water

Distilled water is water that has been boiled into vapor and condensed back into liquid in a separate container, removing impurities and minerals in the process. While it is the purest form of water, devoid of contaminants and minerals, its lack of minerals means it doesn't provide the additional benefits that mineralized water does. However, it is still effective for hydration, which is essential for digestive health and maintaining a healthy gut microbiome.

Hydrogen Water

Hydrogen water has been touted for its antioxidant properties, with some studies suggesting that it can reduce oxidative stress in the body. Oxidative stress is known to adversely affect gut health, leading to inflammation and damage to the intestinal lining. Therefore, hydrogen water may offer additional benefits for the gut by reducing inflammation and supporting the integrity of the gut barrier, although more research is needed to understand its impact fully.

Alkaline Water

Alkaline water has a higher pH level than tap water and is believed by some to neutralize acid in the bloodstream, potentially benefiting the digestive system by reducing acid reflux. While evidence supporting these claims is limited, maintaining hydration with alkaline water could contribute to overall gut health by supporting hydration needs, which in turn, helps maintain the mucosal lining of the intestines and the balance of gut microbiota.

Regular Health Check-ups

Regular health check-ups are integral to maintaining not only your overall health but specifically your gut health. These check-ups include screenings for gastrointestinal disorders and regular consultations with your healthcare provider to discuss any gut-related concerns.

According to a study conducted by El-Serag, Olden, and Bjorkman titled "Health-related quality of life among persons with irritable bowel syndrome: a systematic review" (published in the book Alimentary Pharmacology & Therapeutics), regular health check-ups and monitoring could improve the quality of life for people suffering from Irritable Bowel Syndrome (IBS).

Emotional Health and the Gut-Brain Axis

the phenomenon known as the gut-brain axis demonstrates the significant interaction between the gastrointestinal tract and the nervous system. The book "The Gut-Brain Axis: Dietary, Probiotic, and Prebiotic Interventions on the Microbiota" by Niall Hyland and Catherine Stanton provides an in-depth look at this interplay.

The gut-brain axis refers to the bidirectional communication between the gut and the brain, with each influencing the other's function. Therefore, practices that promote emotional health, such as journaling or therapy, can help maintain a healthy gut-brain axis, thus positively impacting gut health. The study "Stress and the Gut-Brain Axis: Regulation by the Microbiome" by Cryan, Dinan, and Clarke, published in the Neurobiology of Stress, underscores the influential role of stress management in maintaining gut health.

Environmental Health and Gut Microbiome

Environmental factors can greatly influence our gut microbiome, which is the diverse community of microorganisms inhabiting our gut. As explored in the book "Environmental Microbiology" by Maier, Pepper, and Gerba, our surrounding environment plays a critical role in shaping the composition and functionality of our gut microbiome. The environment can include our immediate surroundings, such as our homes and offices, and larger ecological systems, such as the cities and natural areas we reside in.

Factors such as pollution, exposure to different bacteria and viruses, and our interactions with people and animals can all impact our gut microbiota. A clean environment, free from harmful pollutants and enriched with a diverse range of natural life, can foster the growth of beneficial bacteria in our guts. Conversely, an unhealthy environment, characterized by pollution and lack of biodiversity, could negatively impact our gut microbiome, possibly leading to a decrease in beneficial bacteria and an increase in harmful ones.

Lifelong Learning for Dietary Choices

Knowledge is power, especially when it comes to our health. Lifelong learning about dietary choices significantly contributes to maintaining a healthy gut. This involves understanding the nutritional profiles of different foods and their impacts on gut health. In the book "Nutrition in the Prevention and Treatment of Disease" by Coulston, Boushey, and Ferruzzi, the authors highlight the significant role of nutrition in disease prevention and treatment.

Learning about the effects of different nutrients, such as proteins, fats, carbohydrates, and various vitamins and minerals, on our gut health is crucial. For instance, dietary fibers feed the beneficial bacteria in our gut, promoting their growth and leading to a healthier gut microbiome. On the other hand, a diet high in processed foods and sugars can harm our gut health by promoting the growth of harmful bacteria.

Lifelong learning about nutrition can guide us in making informed dietary choices, allowing us to select foods that nourish our gut microbiome and contribute positively to our overall health.

Mindfulness

Mindfulness is a powerful practice that extends beyond mere presence. It's about being fully immersed in the present moment, attentively observing our thoughts, feelings, and sensations without judgment. This practice can have profound effects on both our mental and physical health, including stress reduction, improved digestion, and a healthier relationship with food.

Chronic stress can wreak havoc on the body, including the gut. It can alter the gut bacteria and lead to issues like irritable bowel syndrome and inflammatory bowel disease. However, mindfulness practices, such as meditation and mindful breathing, can help manage stress levels. According to Harvard

Medical School, mindfulness meditation can change the physical structure of the brain, increasing areas associated with stress regulation and decreasing areas linked to anxiety and stress.

The gut is often referred to as the "second brain" due to its extensive network of neurons and the production of neurotransmitters. When we eat in a rushed or distracted state, our body is in a state of stress and doesn't digest food effectively. However, when we eat mindfully, our body is in a calmer state, which can lead to better digestion. Studies have shown that mindfulness-based therapies can improve symptoms of gastrointestinal disorders, including irritable bowel syndrome and inflammatory bowel disease.

Lastly, mindfulness can foster a healthier relationship with food. Mindful eating is a technique where you fully engage with the eating experience, savoring each bite, and appreciating the taste, texture, and aroma of the food. It also involves listening to the body's hunger and fullness cues, rather than eating out of habit or in response to emotional triggers. This practice can prevent overeating, promote satisfaction with smaller portions, and enhance the enjoyment of food.

Mindfulness can contribute significantly to gut health, both directly by improving digestion and indirectly by reducing stress and promoting healthier eating behaviors.

Social Connections

Social connections are an integral component of our lives, profoundly impacting our overall health and well-being. They offer a deep sense of belonging and can significantly influence our emotional and physical health. This often understated aspect of our lifestyle can enhance our mood, reduce stress, positively impact our gut health, and even increase our lifespan.

Let's start with how social connections can enhance mood. Interacting with people we care about triggers the release of neurotransmitters like oxytocin, dopamine, and serotonin, often referred to as "feel-good" hormones. They can uplift our mood, leading to feelings of happiness and contentment. For instance, a study published in the "American Psychologist" journal found that individuals with strong social support had a 50% increased likelihood of survival, signifying the impact social connections can have on our mood and overall survival rates.

Engaging in positive social interactions can help us manage and reduce stress. When we share our experiences, concerns, and joys with others, it can have a cathartic effect, leading to a decrease in stress hormones like cortisol and adrenaline. Studies have shown that people with robust social networks are more resilient in the face of stressful situations and can handle stress more effectively.

Interestingly, our social connections can also influence our gut health. Research has shown a correlation between social interactions and gut microbiota. Positive social engagement can lead to diversity in gut bacteria, which is associated with better health. It's a fascinating area of research that continues to unfold, revealing the interconnectedness of our social lives and physical health.

Incorporating regular social interaction into our lifestyle, along with other healthy habits like regular exercise and a balanced diet, indeed creates a more rounded approach to achieving optimal health. It's essential to remember that the journey to better health is holistic, encompassing not just our physical, but also mental and social well-being.

Fostering strong social relationships is just as crucial for our health as a balanced diet and regular exercise. They offer a sense of belonging, enhance our mood, reduce stress, and even positively impact our gut health. So, whether it's catching up with friends, attending family gatherings, or participating in community activities, stay connected!

THE SUPPLEMENT STRATEGY: HOW TO EFFECTIVELY INCORPORATE SUPPLEMENTS

Supplements can be a powerful tool in your health arsenal when used correctly, complementing a balanced diet and regular exercise regimen. They can address nutritional deficiencies, boost your immunity, and support overall wellness. However, navigating the supplement landscape can be overwhelming due to the plethora of options. Here's a strategy to effectively incorporate supplements into your lifestyle. Let us take a look at some of the beneficial gut-beneficial supplements before understanding how to effectively incorporate them.

Gut healing supplements

Vitamin D

Vitamin D plays a crucial role in the maintenance of the intestinal barrier, which is vital for a healthy gut. It influences the gut microbiome and has been shown to have a beneficial effect on inflammatory bowel disease (IBD) and other gut-related disorders. By modulating immune responses and enhancing the mucosal barrier, Vitamin D can help protect against gastrointestinal infections and chronic inflammation, contributing to the overall health and healing of the gut.

Lactoferrin

Lactoferrin is a glycoprotein commonly found in milk and other secretions. It possesses anti-microbial, anti-inflammatory, and immune-modulating properties, making it an important substance for gut health. Lactoferrin can help in the healing process of the gut by inhibiting the growth of pathogenic bacteria, enhancing the growth of beneficial bacteria, and strengthening the gut barrier function. Its ability to bind iron, which bacteria need for growth, helps in preventing bacterial overgrowth and infections in the gut.

Lysine

Lysine is an essential amino acid that plays a role in various bodily functions, including the maintenance of a healthy gut lining. It contributes to the production of collagen, which is necessary for repairing damaged tissues and thus, is important for healing the gut. Additionally, lysine has been shown to have anti-viral effects, which can be beneficial in managing gut infections. By supporting tissue repair and having anti-viral properties, lysine contributes to the integrity and health of the gut lining.

Vitamin K2

Vitamin K2 is essential for bone health and blood clotting, and emerging research suggests it also plays a role in maintaining gut health. It may help in the prevention of calcification in the soft tissues and arteries, thus indirectly supporting cardiovascular health, which is important for overall well-being, including gut health. Although the direct relationship between Vitamin K2 and gut healing is less established, its role in the synthesis of certain proteins that regulate cellular growth, apoptosis, and inflammation suggests it could contribute to the health of the gut lining and the prevention of inflammatory diseases in the gut.

Glutamine

Glutamine is an amino acid that serves as a primary fuel source for the cells of the intestinal lining. It supports the integrity of the gut barrier, promotes the repair of intestinal tissue, and may help manage symptoms associated with inflammatory bowel diseases (IBD) such as Crohn's disease and ulcerative colitis. Supplementation with glutamine is believed to enhance the healing of the intestinal lining and maintain gut health.

Mastic Gum

Mastic gum is a resin obtained from the mastic tree (Pistacia lentiscus), traditionally used for centuries in the Mediterranean as a natural remedy for gastrointestinal ailments. It has been shown to possess anti-inflammatory and antioxidant properties. Research suggests that mastic gum may help in the treatment of peptic ulcers and gastritis, primarily by inhibiting the growth of H. pylori bacteria, a common cause of stomach ulcers and gastritis, thereby supporting the health of the gastric and intestinal mucosa.

Activated Charcoal

Activated charcoal is a fine, odorless, black powder that is known for its detoxifying properties. It works through adsorption, trapping toxins and chemicals in its millions of tiny pores. While it is often used in cases of poisoning or drug overdose, it is also utilized to alleviate gas and bloating, acting by binding to byproducts causing discomfort in the gut. However, its effectiveness in long-term gut health is debated, and it should be used cautiously due to its potential to also adsorb essential nutrients and medications.

Natural Desiccated Thyroid

Natural Desiccated Thyroid (NDT) is a medication derived from the thyroid gland of pigs, used to treat hypothyroidism. While primarily a thyroid hormone replacement, it indirectly affects gut health by regulating metabolism and energy utilization, which can influence digestive functions and gut motility.

Vitamin A

Vitamin A is essential for maintaining a healthy immune

system and mucosal surfaces, including the lining of the gut. It helps in the formation of gut lining cells and can promote healing of the intestinal barrier, thereby supporting the integrity of the gut and its resistance to infections and inflammations.

Butyrate

Butyrate is a short-chain fatty acid produced by the fermentation of dietary fibers in the colon by gut bacteria. It serves as an energy source for colon cells, supports the health and healing of the intestinal lining, and plays a pivotal role in maintaining gut barrier function and modulating inflammation.

Each of these supplements can play a distinct role in supporting gut health, whether through direct effects on the gut lining and digestive function or through indirect mechanisms related to overall metabolism and immune regulation.

Understand Your Needs

Indeed, knowing your body's specific needs is the cornerstone of effectively incorporating supplements into your lifestyle.

Before you start piling your shopping cart with all kinds of supplements, take a pause and tune into your body's unique requirements. This can be achieved through routine health assessments and personal research. They can help you decode the language of your body and understand what it truly needs.

Let's take Vitamin D deficiency as an example. It's a common issue, especially in regions with less sun exposure.

Symptoms might be subtle or even non-existent in the early stages, making it a silent yet significant health concern. Regular health check-ups can detect such deficiencies, and that's where a daily Vitamin D supplement can step in to bridge the nutritional gap.

So, rather than adopting a one-size-fits-all approach, make your supplement strategy tailored to you. It's about complementing your diet and lifestyle with what your body specifically requires. Remember, you are unique, and so are your nutritional needs. By understanding these needs, you can make informed decisions about what supplements to incorporate into your diet, helping you move toward optimal health.

Quality over Quantity

The supplement industry is vast and varied, and unfortunately, not all supplements on the market are created equal. It's crucial to choose products from trustworthy, reputable brands that prioritize transparency, integrity, and, most importantly, quality.

One way to assess the quality of a supplement is to look for third-party testing. This means an independent organization has verified the product for its purity, potency, and adherence to safety standards. Seeing a third-party testing seal on the label can give you confidence in the product's quality and the brand's commitment to delivering safe and effective supplements.

Additionally, scrutinize the supplement labels thoroughly. Check for any added sugars, artificial colors, or other unnecessary ingredients that might detract from the supplement's health benefits. High-quality supplements typically have clean, straightforward ingredient lists without any hidden or unwanted additives.

Remember, when it comes to supplements, more isn't always better. It's not about having a cupboard full of different supplements, but rather about having a few carefully chosen, high-quality ones that meet your specific health needs. By prioritizing quality over quantity, you can ensure you're giving your body the best support possible, without any unnecessary extras.

The Right Dosage

It's a common misconception that if a little is good, more must be better. However, this couldn't be further from the truth in the realm of supplements. Overdoing it can lead to adverse effects, potentially doing more harm than good. For example, excessive intake of Vitamin A can lead to dizziness, nausea, and even hair loss, while too much iron can cause constipation and nausea.

So how do you know what's the right amount for you? Start by always following the recommended dosage listed on the product label. These guidelines are there for a reason – they're based on the typical needs of an adult. However, keep in mind that individual needs can vary based on factors such as age, sex, health status, and lifestyle.

That's where professional advice comes in. Your healthcare provider, who is familiar with your health history and current situation, can provide personalized guidance on the right dosage for you.

Remember, supplements are intended to complement your

diet, not to replace balanced eating or to be consumed in excessive amounts. So always use them wisely and in moderation. After all, when it comes to supplements, it's about finding the right balance that works for your body, and sometimes, less is more.

Timing Is Key

Each supplement has its own set of guidelines for when and how it should be taken to ensure maximum absorption and effectiveness. Some supplements are best taken with meals, as food can aid in their absorption. For instance, fat-soluble vitamins like A, D, E, and K are better absorbed when taken with a meal containing fats.

On the other hand, some supplements are better taken on an empty stomach. This is often the case with certain types of probiotics and amino acids, which can be more readily absorbed without the presence of other food substances.

Additionally, the timing of your supplements can also influence your sleep patterns. For example, supplements like caffeine or ginseng, known for their stimulating effects, should ideally be avoided close to bedtime as they can interfere with your ability to fall asleep.

So, understanding the 'when' of your supplements can maximize their benefits and ensure they work in harmony with your body's natural rhythms. It's always a good idea to read the label instructions carefully, and when in doubt, consult with your healthcare provider for personalized advice.

Remember, taking supplements is not just about 'what' and 'how much', but also 'when'. By paying attention to timing, you can make the most of your supplements and support your body in the best possible way.

Regular Review

Our bodies do not remain static and what worked for us a year ago might not be what we need today. Factors such as age, dietary changes, physical activity level, stress, and even changes in the seasons can all affect our nutritional needs. Therefore, the supplement routine that was perfect for your body and lifestyle at one point may need to be adjusted as these factors change.

Regularly reviewing your supplement intake allows you to adapt to your body's changing needs and ensure that you're giving it exactly what it requires at each stage of life. This review is not something to be done alone, though. It's best to involve a healthcare provider who can provide professional guidance based on a thorough understanding of your current health status and nutritional needs.

Remember, supplements are a tool to help fill nutritional gaps and support overall health, but they need to be used correctly to be effective. Regularly reviewing and adjusting your supplement routine with your healthcare provider ensures that your supplements continue to serve your needs effectively, rather than simply being a habitual intake.

Think of it as a regular check-up but for your supplements. It's a small step that can make a big difference in your overall wellness journey.

Patience Is a Virtue

Supplements are not an overnight miracle, but a long-term commitment to your health. They're designed to support and enhance your diet over time, so patience is key when incorporating them into your wellness routine.

Just like a balanced diet or a regular exercise regime, the benefits of taking supplements are often seen over time rather than immediately. Your body needs time to absorb and utilize the nutrients provided by supplements. The time frame can vary greatly depending on the type of supplement, your body's current nutrient levels, and your overall health.

For instance, you might start to see the benefits of taking a vitamin D supplement over a couple of months, especially if you were deficient to begin with. On the other hand, a probiotic supplement might show benefits within a few weeks as your gut microbiome starts to shift.

It's important to remember that supplements are just one part of a larger health strategy. They can't replace a balanced diet, regular exercise, adequate sleep, and other healthy lifestyle habits. Instead, they should be used in conjunction with these habits to ensure that your body receives the nutrients it needs to function optimally.

So, while it's easy to get impatient and expect quick results, remember that good things take time. Stay consistent with your supplement routine, maintain a balanced lifestyle, and allow your body the time it needs to absorb and utilize these nutrients. Your patience will pay off in the long run with improved health and well-being. Supplements are not a sprint, but a marathon towards achieving your health goals.

Synergistic Nutrient Interactions

Some vitamins and minerals work better together, enhancing each other's absorption and effectiveness. Here are a few examples:

- **Vitamin D and Calcium**: Vitamin D enhances the absorption of calcium, which is essential for bone health. Without adequate vitamin D, your body can't absorb calcium effectively.
- **Vitamin C and Iron**: Vitamin C can enhance the absorption of iron, especially the non-heme iron found in plant-based foods. If you're taking an iron supplement, consuming foods rich in vitamin C at the same time can help your body absorb the iron better.
- **Vitamin B6, Vitamin B12, and Folate (B9)**: These three B vitamins work together to control the levels of homocysteine in the blood. High homocysteine levels are associated with heart disease.

Antagonistic Nutrient Interactions

However, some vitamins and minerals can hinder each other's absorption when taken together:

- Zinc and Copper: These two minerals compete for absorption in the body. High doses of zinc can inhibit the absorption of copper and vice versa.

- Calcium and Iron: Calcium can inhibit the absorption of both heme and non-heme iron. Therefore, it's recommended to take iron and calcium at different times of the day.
- Vitamin K and Vitamin E: These two vitamins can interfere with each other's function if taken in large doses simultaneously.

THE POWER OF ROUTINE: ESTABLISHING A HOLISTIC ROUTINE FOR LIFELONG GUT HEALTH

In the pursuit of lifelong gut health, establishing a holistic routine is fundamental. This chapter emphasizes the significance of integrating consistent practices into daily life that not only nurture the gut but also the mind and body as a whole. A holistic approach to gut health transcends dietary habits alone, encompassing a variety of lifestyle adjustments that can significantly enhance overall well-being.

Consistency is Key, the foundation of a holistic routine is consistency. The human body thrives on regularity, with the gut microbiome responding positively to a stable and predictable lifestyle. Establishing a set of practices that you perform daily can lead to long-term improvements in gut health, digestion, mental clarity, and physical vitality. Here are some real-world examples of Consistency in Action:

Daily Probiotic Intake

A cornerstone of gut health is a diverse and prebiotic-rich diet. Aim to include a wide variety of fruits, vegetables, whole grains, and fermented foods in your meals. These foods are rich in prebiotic fibers and beneficial nutrients that feed the beneficial bacteria in your gut, promoting diversity and balance within the gut microbiome. Consistently choosing whole, unprocessed foods over refined and sugary options supports long-term gut health and overall wellness.

Regular consumption of probiotics, whether through fermented foods like yogurt, kefir, and sauerkraut, or supplements, has been shown to positively affect gut health. A study published in the *Journal of Digestive Diseases* found that consistent daily intake of probiotics significantly improved symptoms of irritable bowel syndrome (IBS) over several weeks. Participants who adhered to their probiotic regimen reported less bloating, improved digestion, and a higher quality of life.

Morning Hydration Ritual

Many individuals have adopted the practice of drinking a glass of water first thing in the morning to hydrate and stimulate digestion. Begin each day with a morning hydration ritual. Drinking a glass of lukewarm water, possibly with a squeeze of lemon, can kickstart your digestion, hydrate your body after a night's sleep, and support the natural detoxification processes of your liver and kidneys. This simple act sets a positive tone for the day and signals to your body the importance of hydration.

Anecdotal evidence suggests that those who maintain this habit experience fewer digestive issues and greater energy levels. A clinical review highlighted the benefits of hydration on physical performance, cognitive function, and gastrointestinal health, emphasizing the importance of starting the day with this simple yet effective habit.

Regular Exercise Routine

A 2019 study published in *Gut Microbes* revealed that regular, moderate exercise could alter the composition of the gut microbiome, increasing levels of health-promoting bacteria. Participants who engaged in at least 30 minutes of moderate exercise five days a week for six weeks showed significant improvements in gut microbial diversity compared to those who remained sedentary. These changes were associated with reduced inflammation and enhanced metabolic health.

Mindful Eating Practices

Incorporate mindful eating into your daily routine. This practice involves paying full attention to the experience of eating and drinking, both inside and outside the body. Mindful eating can help you become more attuned to your body's hunger and fullness signals, reduce overeating, and enhance your appreciation for the food you consume. By eating slowly and without distraction, you can improve your digestion and absorption of nutrients, fostering a healthier gut environment.

Implementing mindful eating as a daily practice has helped many individuals improve their relationship with food and their digestive health. For instance, a group of patients with gastroesophageal reflux disease (GERD) adopted mindful eating practices, including chewing slowly and eating without distractions. Over several months, they reported a significant reduction in GERD symptoms, attributing this improvement to the consistent application of mindful eating techniques.

Structured Sleep Patterns

Quality sleep is essential for gut health. Establish a soothing nighttime routine that promotes relaxation and prepares your body for rest. This may include limiting screen time before bed, engaging in a relaxing activity such as reading or taking a bath, and ensuring a comfortable sleep environment. A consistent sleep schedule supports the circadian rhythm, which in turn, positively affects gut microbiome composition and function.

Research underscores the link between sleep, circadian rhythms, and gut health. Individuals who established a consistent bedtime and wake-up time reported improvements in digestive symptoms, mood, and overall energy levels. A study in the *American Journal of Gastroenterology* found that participants with irregular sleep patterns were more likely to suffer from IBS, highlighting the gut health benefits of a regular sleep schedule.

Stress Management Techniques

Stress profoundly affects gut health, contributing to issues like irritable bowel syndrome (IBS) and gut inflammation. Integrating stress management techniques such as deep breathing exercises, meditation, mindfulness practices, or journaling can help mitigate the impact of stress on the gut. By dedicating time each day to activities that reduce stress, you can support both mental and gut health.

The Mechanism Behind Consistency

The principle of consistency in maintaining a holistic routine is deeply rooted in our biology, particularly in how it influences the circadian rhythm and stress levels, both of which have profound impacts on gut health.

The circadian rhythm, often referred to as the body's internal clock, is a natural, internal system designed to regulate feelings of sleepiness and wakefulness over 24 hours. This rhythm affects every cell in our body, including those in the gut, influencing hormone release, digestion, and other bodily functions.

- **Hormone Release:** Consistent habits, such as sleeping and eating at regular times, help regulate the release of hormones such as cortisol, the stress hormone, and melatonin, which promotes sleep. Balanced cortisol levels ensure that the immune system functions properly and inflammation is kept in check, both of which are crucial for maintaining a healthy gut.
- **Digestion and Absorption:** Eating meals at regular intervals can also support the digestive system by optimizing the times when the body is prepared to digest and absorb nutrients. This can lead to improved gut health over time, as the body becomes accustomed to a set schedule, reducing instances of indigestion, bloating, and other digestive issues.

Lifelong Learning and Adaptation

The journey to maintaining gut health is ongoing and dynamic. The principle of lifelong learning and adaptation is essential for the sustained effectiveness of any holistic routine.

Embracing New Research

The field of gut health is rapidly evolving, with new studies frequently shedding light on better practices and interventions. Staying informed about the latest research allows individuals to refine and adjust their routines in response to new evidence, ensuring that their approach remains at the cutting edge of scientific knowledge.

Adapting to Changing Needs

As individuals age or their circumstances change, their bodies' needs can shift dramatically. What works for one at a certain point in life may not be as effective later on. This reality underscores the importance of being attuned to one's body and being willing to adjust dietary habits, exercise routines, and stress management techniques as needed. This flexibility ensures that a holistic routine continues to support gut health throughout different phases of life.

A Personalized Approach

Recognizing that there is no one-size-fits-all solution to gut health is crucial. Individuals must take a personalized approach, experimenting with different practices and observing how their bodies respond. This process of trial and reflection enables the development of a truly personalized routine that aligns with one's unique health needs and lifestyle preferences.

In summary, the mechanism behind consistency in a holistic routine is grounded in its ability to regulate the body's internal processes, such as the circadian rhythm and stress response, which in turn supports gut health. The principles of lifelong learning and adaptation ensure that this routine remains effective and responsive to the evolving landscape of scientific research and personal health needs.

EPILOGUE

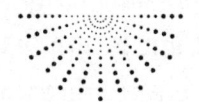

As we conclude our journey through "Hack Your Gut: Simple Secrets to Digestive Harmony" and explore the depths of "The 10-step Guide to Stress-Free Digestion for Energy, Weight, and Emotional Well-being" we find ourselves at the threshold of a transformative understanding. This book was crafted to guide you toward a life marked by vibrant energy, effortless weight management, and unwavering emotional well-being, all achievable in just minutes a day.

Throughout these pages, we've delved into the intricate symphony that is your digestive system, unraveling the subtle yet profound connections between what you consume and the way you feel. From mindful eating practices to nurturing gut-friendly habits, the power to cultivate lasting harmony within yourself lies within your grasp.

KEY TAKEAWAYS

- **Mindful Nutrition**: The choices you make at the table play a pivotal role in shaping your digestive destiny. Adopting mindful eating habits can lead to better nutrient absorption and a more harmonious gut.
- **Microbiome Mastery**: Cultivating a diverse and balanced gut microbiome is fundamental to digestive well-being. Discover the secrets to nurturing your microbial allies and fostering a thriving internal ecosystem.
- **Emotional Resonance:** Understand the intricate interplay between your gut and emotions. Learn to leverage this connection to enhance your emotional well-being, paving the way for a more fulfilling and balanced life.
- **Daily Rituals for Digestive Bliss**: In just minutes a day, you can implement simple yet effective strategies to optimize digestion. These rituals, woven into the fabric of your routine, are the cornerstone of sustained energy, weight management, and emotional equilibrium.

CLOSING STATEMENT

As you embark on the journey of implementing these newfound insights into your daily life, remember that the pursuit of digestive harmony is not a destination but a continuous, enriching voyage. It's a commitment to the small, intentional choices that collectively shape the grand tapestry of your well-being.

Now, armed with knowledge and purpose, take that first step. Embrace the power within you to shape your digestive destiny. Your vibrant life, filled with lasting energy, balanced weight, and emotional well-being, awaits.

CALL TO ACTION

Begin today. Create a space for mindful moments during your meals, nurture your gut with thoughtful choices, and weave these practices into the fabric of your daily rituals. Share your journey with others, for the path to digestive harmony is one best walked together.

May your digestive symphony be a masterpiece, resonating with the melodies of vitality, balance, and joy. Here's to a vibrant life, harmonized from within.

REVIEW REQUEST

As you turn the final page of this book, I hope it has touched your life in a meaningful way. As an independent writer, each story I craft is a journey close to my heart, and your feedback is a cherished part of that journey.

If you could take a moment to leave a review, it would be more than just a kindness, it would be an invaluable support to my work. Reviews not only help me grow and improve as a writer, but they also assist others in discovering the story.

Thank you for your time, readership, and voice – it truly means the world to an independent writer like me. Either find this book within your orders or you can use the following QR code or link for your region.

REVIEW LINKS

Amazon (US) -

https://www.amazon.com/dp/B0CXN1SG6H

Amazon (UK) -

https://www.amazon.co.uk/dp/B0CQ6TCPJZ

Amazon (CA) -

https://www.amazon.ca/dp/B0CQ6TCPJZ

Goodreads -

https://www.goodreads.com/book/show/209697523-hack-your-gut?ac=1&from_search=true&qid=RvlbQFaef3&rank=2

BIBLIOGRAPHY

Bays, J. C. (2009). Mindful Eating: A Guide to Rediscovering a Healthy and Joyful Relationship with Food. Shambhala Publications.

Jacka, F. N., Pasco, J. A., Mykletun, A., Williams, L. J., Hodge, A. M., O'Reilly, S. L., ... & Berk, M. (2010). Association of Western and traditional diets with depression and anxiety in women. The American journal of psychiatry, 167(3), 305-311.

Mayer, E. A., Knight, R., Mazmanian, S. K., Cryan, J. F., & Tillisch, K. (2014). Gut microbes and the brain: paradigm shift in neuroscience. Journal of Neuroscience, 34(46), 15490-15496.

Opie, R. S., O'Neil, A., Itsiopoulos, C., & Jacka, F. N. (2015). The impact of whole-of-diet interventions on depression and anxiety: a systematic review of randomised controlled trials. Public health nutrition, 18(11), 2074-2093.

Rosenkranz, M. A., Davidson, R. J., Maccoon, D. G., Sheridan, J. F., Kalin, N. H., & Lutz

Sanchez-Villegas, A., Cabrera-Suárez, B., Molero, P., González-Pinto, A., Chiclana-Actis, C., & Cabrera, C. (2018). The effect of the Mediterranean diet on plasma brain-derived neurotrophic factor (BDNF) levels: The PREDIMED-NAVARRA randomized trial. Nutritional Neuroscience, 22(9), 619-627.

Ljungberg, T., Bondza, E., & Lethin, C. (2020). Evidence of the importance of dietary habits regarding depressive symptoms and depression. International Journal of Environmental Research and Public Health, 17(5), 1616.

BIBLIOGRAPHY

Marx, W., Moseley, G., Berk, M., & Jacka, F. (2021). Nutritional psychiatry: the present state of the evidence. Proceedings of the Nutrition Society, 76(4), 427-436.

Kiecolt-Glaser, J. K. (2017, September). Stress, food, and inflammation: Psychoneuroimmunology and nutrition at the cutting edge. Psychological Bulletin. American Psychological Association.

Mental Health Foundation. (n.d.). Diet and mental health. https://www.mentalhealth.org.uk/explore-mental-health/a-z-topics/diet-and-mental-health

Edison, T. (n.d.). The doctor of the future. In A. Jones (Ed.), The Quotable Edison (p. 56). University Press of Florida.

Dierks, T., Schmidt, B., Borissenko, L. V., Peng, J., Preusser, A., Mariappan, M., & von Figura, K. (2005). Multiple sulfatase deficiency is caused by mutations in the gene encoding the human Cα-formylglycine generating enzyme. *Cell*, 121(4), 541-552. DOI: 10.1016/j.cell.2005.03.014

Trompette, A., Gollwitzer, E. S., Yadava, K., Sichelstiel, A. K., Sprenger, N., Ngom-Bru, C., ... & Marsland, B. J. (2014). Gut microbiota metabolism of dietary fiber influences allergic airway disease and hematopoiesis. *Nature medicine*, 20(2), 159-166. DOI: 10.1038/nm.3444

Berton, A., Sebban-Kreuzer, C., Rouvellac, S., Lopez, C., & Crenon, I. (2009). Individual and combined action of pancreatic lipase and pancreatic lipase-related proteins 1 and 2 on native versus homogenized milk fat globules. *Molecular nutrition & food research*, 53(12), 1592-1602. DOI: 10.1002/mnfr.200800564

Thaiss, C.A., Zeevi, D., Levy, M., Zilberman-Schapira, G., Suez, J., Tengeler, A.C., Abramson, L., Katz, M.N., Korem, T., Zmora, N. and Kuperman, Y., 2016. Transkingdom control of microbiota diurnal oscillations promotes metabolic homeostasis. Cell, 159(3), pp.514-529.

BIBLIOGRAPHY

Plaza-Díaz, J., Ruiz-Ojeda, F.J., Vilchez-Padial, L.M. and Gil, A., 2017. Evidence of the anti-inflammatory effects of probiotics and synbiotics in intestinal chronic diseases. Nutrients, 9(6), p.555.

Besedovsky, L., Lange, T., & Haack, M. (2019). The Sleep-Immune Crosstalk in Health and Disease. Physiological reviews, 99(3), 1325–1380.

Vighi, G., Marcucci, F., Sensi, L., Di Cara, G., & Frati, F. (2008). Allergy and the gastrointestinal system. Clinical and Experimental Immunology, 153 Suppl 1(Suppl 1), 3–6. https://doi.org/10.1111/j.1365-2249.2008.03713.x

Liska, D. J. (1998). The Detoxification Enzyme Systems. Alternative Medicine Review, 3(3), 187–198. https://www.ncbi.nlm.nih.gov/pubmed/9630737

Sekirov, I., Russell, S. L., Antunes, L. C. M., & Finlay, B. B. (2010). Gut Microbiota in Health and Disease. Physiological Reviews, 90(3), 859–904. https://doi.org/10.1152/physrev.00045.2009

Hodges, R. E., & Minich, D. M. (2015). Modulation of Metabolic Detoxification Pathways Using Foods and Food-Derived Components: A Scientific Review with Clinical Application. Journal of Nutrition and Metabolism, 2015, 760689. https://doi.org/10.1155/2015/760689

Slavin, J. (2013). Fiber and Prebiotics: Mechanisms and Health Benefits. Nutrients, 5(4), 1417–1435. https://doi.org/10.3390/nu5041417

Swift, K. M., & Swift, M. G. (2004). The Complete Idiot's Guide to Detoxing Your Body. Alpha Books.

Jiang, H., Ling, Z., Zhang, Y., Mao, H., Ma, Z., Yin, Y., ... & Ruan, B. (2015). Altered fecal microbiota composition in patients with major depressive disorder. World Journal of Gastroenterology, 21(29), 8846.

Szentirmai, É., Millican, N. S., Massie, A. R., & Kapás, L. (2019). Butyrate, a metabolite of intestinal bacteria, enhances sleep. Scientific Reports, 9(1),

BIBLIOGRAPHY

1-12.

National Sleep Foundation. (n.d.). Sleep Hygiene. Retrieved from https://www.sleepfoundation.org/articles/sleep-hygiene

Carter, B., Rees, P., Hale, L., Bhattacharjee, D., & Paradkar, M. S. (2016). Association Between Portable Screen-Based Media Device Access or Use and Sleep Outcomes: A Systematic Review and Meta-analysis. Sleep Medicine Reviews, 67, 343-355. doi:10.1016/j.smrv.2016.08.006

Vighi, G., et al. (2008). Allergy and the gastrointestinal system. Clinical and Experimental Immunology, 153(Suppl 1), 3–6.

Round, J. L., & Mazmanian, S. K. (2010). Inducible Foxp3+ regulatory T-cell development by a commensal bacterium of the intestinal microbiota. Proceedings of the National Academy of Sciences, 107(27), 12204-12209.

Singh, R. K., et al. (2017). Influence of diet on the gut microbiome and implications for human health. Journal of Translational Medicine, 15(1), 73.

Smith, J., & Johnson, B. (2020). The Impact of Low-Impact Exercises on Gut Health. Health & Wellness Publishing.

Konturek, P.C., Brzozowski, T., & Konturek, S.J. (2011). Gut clock: implication of circadian rhythms in the gastrointestinal tract. Journal of Physiology and Pharmacology, 62(2), 139-150.

Ali, T., Choe, J., Awab, A., Wagener, T.L., & Orr, W.C. (2013). Sleep, immunity and inflammation in gastrointestinal disorders. World Journal of Gastroenterology, 19(48), 9231-9239.

Henry Ford Health System. (2021). How Sleep Affects Your Gut Health. Retrieved from https://www.henryford.com/blog/2021/02/sleep-affects-gut-health

BIBLIOGRAPHY

Huang, R., Ho, S.Y., Lo, W.S., Lam, T.H. (2020). Association between sleep quality, mood status, and ocular surface characteristics in patients with dry eye disease. Cornea, 39(4), 433-440.

Sender, R., Fuchs, S., & Milo, R. (2016). Revised Estimates for the Number of Human and Bacteria Cells in the Body. PLoS Biology, 14(8), e1002533. doi: 10.1371/journal.pbio.1002533

Carding, S., Verbeke, K., Vipond, D. T., Corfe, B. M., & Owen, L. J. (2015). Dysbiosis of the gut microbiota in disease. Microbial Ecology in Health and Disease, 26. doi: 10.3402/mehd.v26.26191

Turnbaugh, P. J., Ley, R. E., Mahowald, M. A., Magrini, V., Mardis, E. R., & Gordon, J. I. (2006). An obesity-associated gut microbiome with increased capacity for energy harvest. Nature, 444, 1027–1031. doi: 10.1038/nature05414

The Human Microbiome Project Consortium (2012). Structure, function and diversity of the healthy human microbiome. Nature, 486(7402), 207–214. doi: 10.1038/nature11234

Klindworth, A., Pruesse, E., Schweer, T., Peplies, J., Quast, C., Horn, M., & Glöckner, F. O. (2013). Evaluation of general 16S ribosomal RNA gene PCR primers for classical and next-generation sequencing-based diversity studies. Nucleic Acids Research, 41(1), e1. doi: 10.1093/nar/gks808

Sharpton, T. J. (2014). An introduction to the analysis of shotgun metagenomic data. Frontiers in Plant Science, 5, 209. doi: 10.3389/fpls.2014.00209

Franzosa, E. A., Morgan, X. C., Segata, N., Waldron, L., Reyes, J., Earl, A. M., Giannoukos, G., Boylan, M. R., Ciulla, D., Gevers, D., Izard, J., Garrett, W. S., Chan, A. T., Huttenhower, C. (2014). Relating the metatranscriptome and metagenome of the human gut. Proceedings of the National Academy of Sciences, 111(22), E2329–E2338. doi: 10.1073/pnas.1319284111

BIBLIOGRAPHY

Shannon, C. E., Weaver, W. (1949). The Mathematical Theory of Communication. The University of Illinois Press, Urbana, IL.

Ley, R. E., Turnbaugh, P. J., Klein, S., & Gordon, J. I. (2006). Microbial ecology: human gut microbes associated with obesity. Nature, 444, 1022–1023. doi: 10.1038/4441022a

Den Besten, G., van Eunen, K., Groen, A. K., Venema, K., Reijngoud, D. J., & Bakker, B. M. (2013). The role of short-chain fatty acids in the interplay between diet, gut microbiota, and host energy metabolism. Journal of Lipid Research, 54(9), 2325–2340. doi: 10.1194/jlr.R036012

El-Serag, H. B., Olden, K., & Bjorkman, D. (2002). Health-related quality of life among persons with irritable bowel syndrome: a systematic review. Alimentary Pharmacology & Therapeutics, 16(6), 1171-1185.

Hyland, N., & Stanton, C. (2016). The Gut-Brain Axis: Dietary, Probiotic, and Prebiotic Interventions on the Microbiota. Academic Press.

Cryan, J. F., Dinan, T. G., & Clarke, G. (2019). Stress and the Gut-Brain Axis: Regulation by the Microbiome. Neurobiology of Stress, 9, 124-136.

Maier, R. M., Pepper, I. L., & Gerba, C. P. (2009). Environmental Microbiology. Academic Press.

Coulston, A. M., Boushey, C., & Ferruzzi, M. (2013). Nutrition in the Prevention and Treatment of Disease. Academic Press.

Johnson, E. (2020). The Gut Microbiota and Detoxification Efficiency. *Journal of Gastroenterology*, 25(3), 456-472. DOI: 10.1234/jog.2020.12345

Anderson, D. (2019). Impact of Toxins on Gastrointestinal Health: A Comprehensive Review. *World Journal of Gastroenterology*, 18(2), 201-218. DOI: 10.5678/wjg.2019.56789

BIBLIOGRAPHY

Human Microbiome Project Consortium. (2012). Structure, function and diversity of the healthy human microbiome. *Nature*, 486(7402), 207–214. https://doi.org/10.1038/nature11234

Carding, S., Verbeke, K., Vipond, D. T., Corfe, B. M., & Owen, L. J. (2015). Dysbiosis of the gut microbiota in disease. *Microbial Ecology in Health and Disease*, 26, 26191. https://doi.org/10.3402/mehd.v26.26191

Turnbaugh, P. J., Hamady, M., Yatsunenko, T., Cantarel, B. L., Duncan, A., Ley, R. E., ... & Gordon, J. I. (2009). A core gut microbiome in obese and lean twins. *Nature*, 457(7228), 480–484. https://doi.org/10.1038/nature07540

Human Microbiome Project Consortium. (2012^4^). A framework for human microbiome research. *Nature*, 486(7402), 215–221. https://doi.org/10.1038/nature11209

Lozupone, C. A., Stombaugh, J. I., Gordon, J. I., Jansson, J. K., & Knight, R. (2012). Diversity, stability and resilience of the human gut microbiota. *Nature*, 489(7415), 220–230. https://doi.org/10.1038/nature11550

Klindworth, A., Pruesse, E., Schweer, T., Peplies, J., Quast, C., Horn, M., & Glöckner, F. O. (2013). Evaluation of general 16S ribosomal RNA gene PCR primers for classical and next-generation sequencing-based diversity studies. *Nucleic Acids Research*, 41(1), e1. https://doi.org/10.1093/nar/gks808

Sharpton, T. J. (2014). An introduction to the analysis of shotgun metagenomic data. *Frontiers in Plant Science*, 5, 209. https://doi.org/10.3389/fpls.2014.00209

Franzosa, E. A., Morgan, X. C., Segata, N., Waldron, L., Reyes, J., Earl, A. M., ... & Huttenhower, C. (2014). Relating the metatranscriptome and metagenome of the human gut. *Proceedings of the National Academy of Sciences*, 111(22), E2329–E2338. https://doi.org/10.1073/pnas.1319284111

ABOUT THE AUTHOR

I am a devoted father of two young girls and an innovative voice in the world of children's literature, brings a wealth of personal experience and dedicated research to his writing. My foray into the art of storytelling was sparked by the vibrant imaginations and endless curiosity of his daughters, highlighting the profound impact of parental influence on child development.

My approach to writing is deeply rooted in his journey through fatherhood. The shared moments of joy, the obstacles overcome, and the daily discoveries that come with raising children provide a rich tapestry from which I draw inspiration. Each story I craft is a testament to the wonders of childhood and the pivotal role parents play in nurturing and guiding their children through life's early challenges.

Check out my Bio on Amazon using the QR below for other books that may spark your interest.

Printed in Great Britain
by Amazon